The Pilates Path to Health

The Pilates Path to Health Body, Mind, and Spirit

Gary Calderone

Word Keepers, Inc.
Published by Bibliocast
Fort Collins, Colorado

Word Keepers, Inc.
Bibliocast/Sat Nam Imprints/Imagine Books/Hawk's Cry Publications

Books are available at specialty quantity discounts for bulk purchases for promotions, fund-raising, and educational needs.

For details, write or telephone:
Word Keepers, Inc.
Tel. 970-225-8058
Fax 877-445-1007
wordkeepersinc@gmail.com
www.wordkeepersinc.com

Cover/Interior Design: onedesign

Library of Congress Cataloging-in-Publication Data

Calderone, Gary

The pilates path to health/Gary Calderone

Includes bibliographical references.

ISBN-13: 978-0-9795315-8-3
ISBN-10: 0-9795315-8-6

1. Personal growth, life situations, health 2. Joseph Pilates philosophy of Contrology 3. Self-improvement through mind-body connection in Pilates Method 4. Health through exercise 5. Self-awareness (Psychology) (Health) (Philosophy), (Spirituality), etc. 6. Inspiration, heart-warming stories of overcoming physical limitations to healthier lifestyles 7. Body's wisdom (Principles of Biology and Physiology) 8. Pilates Elders, teaching, instruction, training

I. Title

First Bibliocast/Word Keepers, Inc. paperback edition May 2011

Manufactured in the United States of America

"Always consult your physician before beginning any exercise program. This information contained herein is not intended to diagnose any medical condition or to replace your healthcare professional."

10 9 8 7 6 5 4 3 2 1

Dedication

Pilates teachers, students, and enthusiasts

Applause

"It is minds like Calderone's mind that will help speed up the day, where a critical mass will embrace a peaceful and balanced state between body, mind, and spirit hastening the shift in our world's paradigm from one of anger to one of love."

—Brent D. Anderson, P.T., Ph.D., OCS, President and Co-founder of Polestar Pilates

"Because there is so much trendy hype about Pilates it is imperative that the real value of this work be spoken about loudly and creatively as Gary has done in this book. Pilates is transformative."

—Rachel Taylor Segel with **Amy Taylor Alpers,** Co-founder and Co-owner, The Pilates Center Boulder, Colorado

"Gary asks the right questions . . . he illuminates the truth about how choices for our inner health are mirrored in the manifestation of our outer experience, thereby strengthening global consciousness. Truly inspiring!"

—Clare Dunphy, Peak Pilates Master Trainer, Director, Progressive Bodyworks, Inc.

"Anyone who has had the opportunity to read this work will find themselves eagerly awaiting their next Pilates session. I myself feel more 'anchored into my bones, the earth, and my life' just having read the manuscript."

—Zoe Stein Pierce, Director, Pilates at Dancescape Studio, The Premier Pilates Studio of Fort Worth, Texas

"This book is important for the existence and survival of Joseph Pilates intention in the world."

—Lara Kolesar, Master Pilates Teacher

Author's Note

The acquirement and enjoyment of physical well-being, mental calm, and spiritual peace are priceless to their possessors if there be any such so fortunate living among us today. However, it is the ideal to strive for, and in our opinion, it is only through Contrology that this unique trinity of a balanced body, mind, and spirit can ever be attained. —Joseph Pilates (1945)

Gary Calderone's life is a powerful testament to the transformational power of Pilates. Pilates changes lives. It did his, as it has for so many others. With Pilates as his beacon, Gary brought himself back from the brink of debilitating illness. In this timely and richly informative book, Gary shares his inspiring road to recovery, as he traces the century-long journey that has seen Pilates emerge world-wide as one of the most impactful modalities for health, fitness, and healing on the planet. Gary roots his work and philosophy in the foundational work of Joseph Pilates' *Contrology*. The author stands on the backs of Joseph Pilates, the "Elders," and every instructor/student/client before him. Gary Calderone personally recognizes the healing gift of Pilates. Pilates brought him back from illness and a lack of balance in his personal life and life purpose. His life became unified, whole. Healing is an inside job. It is maintenance—the *Contrology*—of self. Most of us are not given an *owner's manual:* We bungle toward balance and health. We rush. We eat and drink too much, too little. We work more and play less. We live outside of our natural selves; holding up; putting off, or just getting through until we can "feel or fix" it later; until we can turn a corner and discover the truth—health is the natural state of the body. Balance is within our grasp. That's the gift of this book: a contemporary voice of who, what, and how we find that balance, that preventative system that seeks liberation from restrictive suffering. "Pilates changes lives!" This echoed true then, and echoes true now. *Contrology* is evolving in global communities seeking balance in all categories of their lives. This book is the marker of how Pilates is adapting and serving a 21st century world.

Table of Contents

Foreword
by Wendy LeBlanc-Arbuckle

Of the millions of people practicing the Pilates Method around the world today, very few know the depth of the vision that inspired Joseph Pilates to create this profound exercise system. In fact, most people still associate Pilates, almost exclusively, with specific exercises performed on mat and spring-based apparatus. Yet, Joseph Pilates was far more than just a purveyor of exercises.

He was a true visionary who taught from a coordinated trinity of body, mind, and spirit. Indeed, his system of Contrology evolved from his lifelong exploration of both ancient and contemporary movement forms, along with the holistic living principles that are at their foundation. For Joseph Pilates, movement was a metaphor for life. His exercises always "lived" for him in a much larger vision . . . that we discover our own inner wisdom, our ability to self-heal and reconnect with the vital forces that constitute our true nature. He was passionate that we come to know that we can live our natural birthright, a life filled with "spontaneous zest and pleasure."

Yet, he saw that in our rush for quick answers to many of life's questions and daily challenges, we often look outside ourselves, becoming increasingly removed from our instinctive wisdom. In looking for answers, rather than being willing to "enter the inquiry" that life is, he saw that we have become increasingly disconnected with that which truly nourishes us.

We don't have to look far to see the truth of the insights he was making more than a half century ago! We have forgotten how breathing naturally nourishes and cleanses the body. We walk in shoes that look good, but don't allow our feet to get stronger and properly support the entire body. We sit in poorly designed chairs for long periods, losing our once intuitive awareness of core balance. We are often unconscious about the daily and seasonal rhythm of eating, the quality of our food, or its balancing (or imbalancing) effect on our bodies. We forget that the spine needs to move in multi-directions, the way children and animals move naturally. Joseph Pilates was clearly ahead of his time.

He understood these contradictions, and took upon himself the formidable task of spreading his vision, and the profound benefits of his system of Contrology, to the masses. Built upon the underlying and governing laws of nature, his brilliant system of movement was always a means to a much greater end . . . living a life full of inspired passion, focused purpose, and abundant vitality!

As a second generation Pilates teacher, this inspired vision has always been at the heart of my exploration into Pilates. And, it is this exploration that called to Gary Calderone, more than a decade ago, to relocate to Austin and immerse himself in my Core Connections® Pilates work—the body of work that has evolved from my lifelong study of the unifying principles that form the foundation of all the great body/mind systems.

As we worked together over these years, I watched Gary's desire to share his deepening awareness of Joseph Pilates' mission grow brighter and brighter. His passion has become contagious and his desire to illuminate and share Joe's vision unwavering.

This book is a culmination of Gary's commitment to expand public awareness, beyond the trappings of the Pilates Fitness Craze, to the true transformational potential of this work.

Joseph Pilates' life was a dramatic reflection of his vision; and now, through this timely and beautifully crafted book, Gary Calderone has given us a window through which we, too, can reflect on an even grander path with our Pilates practice. Whether you are a Pilates teacher, dedicated client, or brand new to Pilates, there is a potent message available in this book. Its message will inspire you, challenge you, and, just maybe, call you forth in a way that unfolds a renewed possibility of living a life that is filled with, in Joe's words, *"the priceless gift of physical well-being, mental calm, and spiritual peace."*

Wendy LeBlanc-Arbuckle
Director of Education, Pilates Center of Austin
Core Connections® Pilates Continuing Education

Preface

I have come to learn that the system of physical exercises, popularly known as Pilates, began to be developed during World War I as a comprehensive *method of physical, mental, and spiritual conditioning called Contrology* by a man who was at that time confined to a British internment camp for the crime of growing up in Germany. His name was Joseph Hubertus Pilates, and only after his death in 1967 did his wife and co-teacher, Clara, begin calling the work 'Pilates' in his honor. Joseph Pilates left us with his legacy. Today, accepted worldwide without division by origin, race, or creed, his philosophy of Contrology, written in R*eturn to Life Through Contrology* (1945) is, as it was then, *a decisive exposition of what his exercises, known today as Pilates, can do for an individual.* So is this 21st century interpretation, *The Pilates Path to Health: Body, Mind, and Spirit,* my expanded exposition of what Pilates has and continues to offer me and what I believe it can offer individuals living in these tumultuous times.

As a Pilates community we—teachers and our students and clients and equipment purveyors—have done much to ensure and preserve the work of Joe and Clara through authenticity, comprehensive training programs, and accreditation, and duplication with some changes of precise measurements for the continued manufacturing of safe and effective Pilates equipment. However, we have not yet *fully recognized, evolved, or applied the entirety and potential of his philosophy as written, on which he built his work, in terms relevant to our modern day.*

This book is the culmination of the author's sixteen-year search for a comprehensive answer to the question: *Why is my life experience, and that of others, greatly enhanced by a Pilates session?* From a primal perspective, it can be said that there are two main motivating factors that keep us living: avoidance of pain and pursuit of pleasure. For the author, Pilates specializes in harmonizing the co-existence of these opposites.

Much of my understanding has come from observing others while teaching the Pilates method, and from countless conversations with clients, teachers, students, and enthusiasts through the years. If those observations were not profound enough, the changes in me certainly were. My personal story is detailed later in this book.

My quest led me to investigate the life of Joseph Pilates, the times during which he came to manhood, and the events and influences that led him to develop the method of health restoration which now bears his name. That story is told in Part One.

Joe Pilates did not name his method for himself. He called his work Contrology, deriving this word from the conviction that the mind can be brought to control the muscles and bones of the body so thoroughly that most, if not all, suffering can be relieved through diligent and persistent use of his method.

In Part Two and following, you will discover, through the stories of Pilates clients and teachers, as well as from the words of Joseph Pilates himself, why this decades-old 'exercise program' that is now sweeping the world can actually be an ideal approach to healing, growth, and transformation of the body-mind. In his original philosophy, his conception of fitness was a prerequisite to achieve happiness. Pilates is even more effective now in closing the gap between painful and pleasurable living with the additional understanding and application of biomechanical knowledge that has become available since Joe's death.

This 21st century interpretation of Pilates Contrology and its underlying philosophy tells a story of how human beings can reach their full potential practicing Pilates, explaining why the decades-old method is so vital and relevant to our lives today. From the teachers, clients, and students I've spoken with throughout the years, I see that there is something we are all intuiting about Pilates—that what we are teaching and learning is more than *just about exercises.* The art and science of *living life to its fullest is the Pilates promise* and was Joe's intention.

If you listen to Madison Avenue's idea of fitness, you might think you need 'six-pack abs' and 'buns of steel'—the beefcake body of a strongman or the willowy but sculpted form of a supermodel. Joe Pilates rarely wrote about any of that, and that's not what this book is about. The goal of Pilates is not a glamorous physique, but rather, a *return to health,* or in Joe's words a *"Return to Life."* This book is based on evidence of outcomes produced by doing Pilates. The evidence herein referred to as the *"unspoken"* benefits, include, but are not limited to: reduction in pain, physical and emotional healing, and a shift in perception and personal paradigm, bringing a heightened state of awareness. This new awareness is obtained from embracing the proven method ('Contrology' for Joe, 'Pilates' for us) which has survived the test of time.

The intention of Joe's Contrology was to move humanity to greater potential through awareness, balance, and self-knowledge—the awareness growing out of the techniques of Contrology extending far beyond mere exercise. Joe was a bit messianic in his conviction that only through Contrology could a unique trinity of body, mind, and spirit be attained. In his experience, ". . . consciousness of possessing the power to accomplish our desires with renewed, lively interest in life is the natural result of the practice of Contrology."

Perhaps the writing of this book—reflecting an affirmation in the Pilates Community that there is greater purpose and wisdom beyond the exercises we do and teach—is timely. It is certainly purposeful timing in my own life, but it may also be in alignment with the needs of a 21st century world. Joe's two books, reflective of his eighty-four years on the planet (1883–1967) and life as it was then, were written in one of the most tumultuous times of global consciousness, or lack thereof, particularly the 30's and 40's. Life today is tempered by a growing sense of the overwhelming challenges we face in national and global affairs. This book is intended to expand internal awareness to better face those challenges—to build on what you know, to illuminate the reason that drives your practice. It is intended to help define what may be elusive or incomplete in your understanding of a coordinated, uniquely balanced trinity of body, mind, and spirit and the impact that has on our lives *today*. It is intended to help support individuals practicing the Pilates method, to support that consciousness Joseph Pilates referred to so many decades ago, to accomplish our desires from a position of renewed life!

It is my understanding and my intention to suggest, based on the context of this book, that the execution of Pilates was Joseph Pilates' hope that people would and could change their way of thinking and their lives to the betterment of humankind by embracing his work. I am a firm believer in the pull of the future—that everything is connected, past, present, and future, and that nothing is happenstance. The surge in the popularity of Pilates, its steady growth around the world, and its future I see as part of a great rethinking—a spectrum of growth in self-awareness and knowledge. Joe, among a few others, brought us back to our bodies, to the importance of taking on working with the body. He gave us the tools to do it. As Carl Jung gave us the tools for an understanding of our whole psyche, or as Ida Rolf gave us tools to experience the structural integration of self. Many play their parts. Joe, for his part, believed that his work would live forever. The day before he died he is known to have said, "Everyone will be doing my method." Not popular in his time except among dancers who knew his value and to those lucky enough to find him, it seems he was right! Pilates is now available all over the world.

Consider this quote from author Russell McDougal from his booklet *The Isle of View: JOB Just Orchestrating Balance:*

Our ongoing job in life is to find a balance with all the needs and challenges we have coming towards us. Life is a dance, and we have to juggle things to find a sense of balance. May we find that center that gives us the balance to find grace and magic of life. Let go of attachments and judgments, and let your mind be in harmony. It's a dance. It's a trance. It's a romance with the balance of life.

News forecasts dark events as if *outside* of our control. Pilates offers the opportunity for a balance—change occurs *inside* you, preparing you to face the challenges of the modern world. Within ourselves, we can discover an area of inner space: a new capacity. Inviting suggestions to *breathe, release, and expand ourselves, helped by* the tactile support of a mat, springs, pulleys, straps, push-bars, barrels, and chairs to conjure up new sensations and to experience what once seemed undoable. Pilates gives you an opportunity to align yourself and open yourself to life's creative spontaneity, as unpredictable and perhaps elusive as that can be. Pilates gives you an opportunity to let go of old patterns and notions to attain an abundance of possibility. I hope this book offers you a greater awareness of how to orchestrate that balance in today's world.

Gary Calderone
Fort Collins, Colorado

Part One

The Life & Times of
Joseph H. Pilates

The Life & Times of Joseph H. Pilates

Truth will prevail and that is why I know my teaching will reach the masses and finally be adopted as universal. —Joseph H. Pilates

History is subjective. Some say, history goes to the victorious; those who win the wars and dominate lands and peoples and cultures, those are the individuals who write our history. Much of what we know today to be historically true is only as accurate as the means by which information was disseminated. What is purported to be historical fact can be blurred or falsified by human error, conjecture, malicious intention, political agenda, and/or legend. This historical overview of the life and times of Joseph Pilates is a *stock* version of what has been passed down through decades of stories, articles, interviews, documents, embellishments, and now my own perceptions of that 'history.'

When history does birth an era of great visionaries like that of Joseph Pilates, humanity benefits, individually and collectively, from their contributions. These icons of personality and persuasion offer alternative choices from the 'norm' of current accepted parameters of the human condition. Information, knowledge, beauty, wisdom, growth, further possibility, and hope are the very least of what humanity can receive. On a grander scale, these 'thinkers outside the box' present a platform of transformation in both *concept* and *the particular.* They are ahead of their time.

Joseph H. Pilates was one such icon, an inventor, philosopher, and visionary. His work has shifted a long-standing view of the fitness paradigm. Even his critics claimed him fifty years ahead of his time. His messages are available in his two books: *Your Health* (1934) and *Return to Life Through Contrology* (1945). His thoughts that validated his methods are as pertinent today as they were then. His premise that the world would improve overall through the health of its people was relevant *then* and is relevant *today.* When we consider these contemporary, tumultuous times and the threats facing humanity then and now (war, pollution, climate changes, population increases, third world living conditions for growing global populations, and growing concerns for clean food and water supplies), we haven't come too far. There is still a need for each individual to participate in self-responsibility, self-healing, self-direction, and self-awareness. Joseph Pilates brought these ideals to the world more than six decades ago.

Joseph Pilates' writings, although informative, are not what are powerful about his work. His messages are best delivered through, as witnessed by those who *get it,* the developmental process and awareness inherent in his prescribed Pilates Method. Avid participants practicing the Pilates Method claim that their lives have changed. This book attempts to contribute to Joseph Pilates' work by affirming that his method and his lifework continues to live on, offering value to the personal lives of individuals practicing the Pilates Method today.

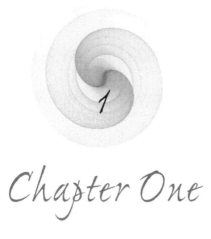

Chapter One

The Early Years

History tells us Joseph Hubertus Pilates was born in 1883 to a German mother and a father of Greek origin in Mönchengladbach, a small town near Dusseldorf. By all accounts he was a sickly child, suffering from asthma, rickets, and a bout of rheumatic fever, among other maladies. His father was a prize-winning gymnast and his mother a naturopath, influences which undoubtedly fed his youthful determination to become physically stronger and helped to instill in him the appreciation for good health and physical development. He and his wife Clara devoted their lives to help others. Their love and partnership culminated in the creation and teaching of the system of physical exercises which now bears his name, the Pilates Method.

Joe would later recount that when a family physician gave him an old anatomy book, "I learned every page, every part of the body. I would move each part as I memorized it." In his quest to find the keys to natural and healthful movement he fed his thirst for knowledge of the body and its wisdom by observing nature, watching animals, especially cats, and studying babies. He quietly observed and learned. He spent hours watching animals move about effortlessly and play in their environment, particularly watching their innate habits upon waking from sleep, taking copious notes on their movements when stretching. From newborn infants and cats, Joe distilled the essence of innocence, now evidenced in the freedom of movement of the Pilates exercises. "I base my method on the baby and the cat," was Joe's comment in an interview he gave in 1959 for a now defunct New York City newspaper. That article seen and read by Mary Bowen, now a Pilates Elder, was what brought her to Joe and Clara in the first place.

Joe also learned by personal experience, sickness, and infirmity to decipher the secrets to healthy life. This, to me, is the most revealing aspect of Joe's legacy. He survived his own decline, conditions that could, in his time, lead to the grave. When Joe reached adolescence, he had become such a model of physical development that he posed for anatomical charts. His commitment to physical fitness and personal development helped him to overcome asthma and rickets, his boyhood frailties. He also went on to become a successful gymnast, boxer, diver, self-defense expert, and circus performer. He remained robustly active until his death in 1967 at the age of eighty-four, *exceeding the standard life expectancy of his time.*

Chapter Two

European Fitness Trends and the Young Muscleman

It is worth noting that Joseph Pilates grew to manhood at a time when 'scientific physical culture' was drawing great attention across Europe, conjuring a general opinion that the mind is the absolute master of the body. Joe's contribution to the development of this notion was that it was the coordinated relationship between the body and mind that created whole body health. His scientific method would inform the renewal of our cells and progressively decrease the suffering of generations to come. By the mid-nineteenth century, Indian yogis had begun visiting Europe and teaching their ancient system, though their influence was at first limited and localized. (It is not known whether Joe personally encountered such teachings from the East.) Joe's method was later recognized as an integration of the influences of Eastern and Western philosophies: Eastern health philosophy meets Western technology. This marriage may be the greatest distinction of the Pilates Method.

The outcome from practicing Joe's method was different than the approach of fitness leaders of his time. According to historical references, Pilates derived his method from multiple disciplines, at least in part. When asked what *any one of these exercises* was good for, his response was, "It's good for the whole body." His response refers to the holistic nature of the execution of Pilates exercises. This distinction identifies the Pilates Method as *different* in inception and execution from general exercise practices.

By the dawn of the 20th century, a 'fitness revolution' had captured the public's imagination in the West, with notable support from such public figures as King George of England and U.S. President William Howard Taft and President Woodrow Wilson.

One such acknowledged leader of this fitness movement was Polish-born physician Vladislav Krayevsky who, in 1885, founded the St. Petersburg Amateur Weightlifting Society. Krayevsky believed that a physical fitness culture was a crucial ingredient in the prevention and treatment of illness. Among his many followers was the famous strongman George Hackenschmidt who credited Krayevsky with teaching him everything he knew. Krayevsky himself published two influential books on physical development at the turn of the century. Joseph Pilates, by then a budding athlete and strongman, as well as an avid reader (it would be assumed) was aware of Krayevsky's teachings.

Another leading advocate of physical fitness culture during the same era was the Russian-born strongman, George

Sandow, who distinguished himself by combining superb physical development with a flair for showmanship, a superb teaching ability, and public generosity. Sandow not only bested other great strongmen of his day, but he was an early champion of hygienic working conditions for the poor, and a tireless promoter of mandatory physical education and sports in public education. So great was his influence, that in 1911 he was appointed Professor of Scientific Physical Culture to His Majesty King George.

The following year, 1912, Joseph Pilates ventured to England, intent on perfecting his skills as a boxer. Like Sandow, he had a flair for showmanship that would serve him well. He soon found work as a gymnast in a traveling circus, and by 1914 was one of the star attractions. Then something happened that would change his life forever.

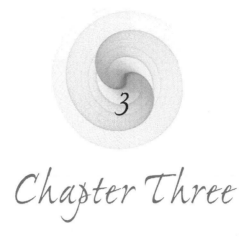

Chapter Three

Turning Point: War and Internment

War broke out between England and Germany, and Joseph Pilates found himself interned at a camp for 'enemy aliens,' first in Lancaster and later on the Isle of Man. Until this time, he had devoted his life to self-improvement and athletic prowess, but now he turned his attention to the health and fitness needs of others. This marked the real beginning of what became his life's work and his legacy. Using equipment evolved from hospital beds, Joe aided in the recovery from affliction, wounds, illness, and infirmity with his ingenious insights on how to *support* the body under *traumatic circumstances*. This profound healthful advantage is *the "unspoken" benefit* of Joseph H. Pilates' legacy today. Before the war was over, he had already laid the foundations of the method he called Contrology, proving its efficacy on fellow inmates of the internment camp.

While at Lancaster, he taught wrestling and self-defense to any who were interested, promising his students they would emerge from their confinement more fit than when they arrived. The biggest breakthrough in the development of his health system came, though, when he was transferred to the forbidding camp at Knockaloe, Patrick, on the Isle of Man. Originally meant to hold 5,000 internees, Knockaloe, by the war's end, held some 24,500, crowded into wooden huts in an area of only twenty-two acres.

Into this squalid situation came Joe Pilates. Before long he became a fixture at the camp hospital, tending scores of bed-ridden men as a self-appointed nurse-physiotherapist. There he began devising makeshift equipment to help rehabilitate those suffering from injuries and the effects of long term confine-ment, drawing on his memory of equipment encountered in his training as a gymnast. Attaching bedsprings to the head-boards and footboards of hospital beds, he created resistance exercises which would later become the spring-based Pilates apparatus, (mainstays of Contrology,) and influence 'state of the art' physical therapy techniques. His patients thrived. (Today these 'beds' have evolved in design to accommodate the needs of chronic illness populations, like Parkinson's Disease, through the innovative techniques applied by Pilates savvy Physical Therapists.)

The Spanish flu epidemic of 1918 killed millions across Europe and was particularly hard on the populations of crowded prison camps. The Pilates fitness regimen apparently made a huge difference at Knockaloe. It is said that not one detainee under his care succumbed to the flu.

When the war ended, Joe returned to Germany and worked for a time as a self-defense and fitness trainer for the Hamburg Military Police. He also continued to develop his exercise machines, which he used to help rehabilitate rheumatic patients. During this time he met Rudolph von Laban, an influential movement analyst who is said to have incorporated some of Pilates' theories into his own work. Joe also taught innovative warm-up exercises to the famous German dancer and choreographer, Mary Wigman, the first of many such artists drawn to his ideas.

Joe was invited to become a physical trainer for the new German army (some biographies say the 'invitation' was actually an order from the Kaiser), but he was uncomfortable with the political direction Germany was taking and decided it was time to leave Germany.

Chapter Four

Contrology, Success, and Celebrity

With the help of boxer Max Schmeling, Joseph Pilates set sail for America. Aboard his ship, he met a woman named Clara, a nurse and kindergarten teacher who was suffering from arthritis. During the voyage, he worked with her to relieve her pain, and by the time they reached New York, they had fallen in love. Legend is unsure as to when or if they married, intent on working together to promote Contrology. Clara quickly became Joe's most capable student and his co-teacher. For the next four decades, they worked side by side, and Clara carried on the work for another decade after Joe's passing.

They took an apartment on Eighth Avenue in New York City and set up the first Pilates Studio there. It was a strategic location; a number of dance studios and rehearsal spaces were located in the same building. Before long, many of New York's best dancers and theatrical performers were coming to the

Pilates Studio. George Balanchine, famed choreographer for the New York City Ballet, studied with Joe and sent many of his dancers to the studio for *strengthening* and *balancing* as well as *rehabilitation*. Modern dance legends Martha Graham and Hanya Holm also became devotees. By 1956, *Dance* magazine could report, "At some time or other virtually every dancer in New York has meekly submitted to the spirited instruction of Joe Pilates."

His exercise routines emphasized the importance of using fewer sets of only a few repetitions of compound movements, which use significant motor skill and coordination, as opposed to the more typical regime of extensive repetition of fairly automatic movements. His rationale for this was that prolonged repetitive routines tend to reduce mental involvement, whereas performance of carefully executed sets of few repetitions of skilled movements affords a better balance of mind-and-body training.

A firm believer in documenting results, Joe was one of the first physical trainers to use before-and-after photographs of his students. Such photo sets leave no doubt that Contrology was getting consistently impressive results in as little as two months of regular sessions. I have seen these photographs, and to say the results were dramatic would be an understatement. Today, in a private session, not only do some teachers choose to take before and after photos as a record of verifiable results, but *notate subjective life changing outcomes that clients experience.*

In recent years there has been discussion and scrutiny whether the ideas for Pilates equipment originated from Joe.

Joe's initiative to develop equipment was by design: to meet client individual needs and improve the ergonomics of sparse living conditions of New York City apartment life. Today this tradition is considered for the development of innovative equipment.

Joe was a thinker and a creator—what stands as distinctive is how Joe put the whole thing together in his special way, along with amazing spring-based apparatus surpassing the standard of his day.

From his first experiments with bed springs during World War I until the end of his life, Joe never tired of creating and perfecting the partnership of machine and method. This equipment was then known as apparatus, and today it is recognized as Pilates equipment i.e. exercise machines that have become synonymous with the Pilates Method. Today these exercise machines help to discern individual physical assessments, measure results, and support pain management.

Joe had a workshop below his Eighth Avenue apartment where he and his brother Fred tinkered endlessly, resulting in such Pilates staples as the Cadillac, the Universal Reformer, the Barrel, and the Wunda Chair. The creative intelligence stimulated from 'tinkering' is the catalyst of many great innovators.

What is apparent is the intrinsic nature of how his method teaches whole body awareness. What is distinct and original about Joseph Pilates' partnership of equipment and method is the repeating component consistently representative in subsequent movements. Practice of the Pilates Method reminds us that we are consciously interactive with the outcome through our participation in our own healthy lifestyle.

Though a legend among professional dancers, Joe did not live to see his life's work become today's household name. His two books, *Your Health* (1934) and *Return to Life Through Contrology* (1945), were well reviewed, but not widely read during his lifetime. He often claimed to be fifty years ahead of his time. Based upon the virtual explosion of interest in his work in just the past decade, it seems he was right.

Chapter Five

Zest to the Last

Joe lived what he taught—that Contrology leads to zestful, happy living through the attainment of a balanced body, mind, and spirit. "Physical fitness is the first requisite of happiness," wrote Joe in *Return to Life Through Contrology*. "Our interpretation of physical fitness is the attainment and maintenance of a uniformly developed body with a sound mind fully capable of naturally, easily, and satisfactorily performing our many and varied daily tasks with spontaneous zest and pleasure." This definition represents the intended outcome of what 21st century vernacular calls a 'workout.' As you can see, our definition of 'workout' broadens to include 'a healthy body' in our understanding of physical fitness and a balance in body, mind, and spirit.

Joe practiced what he preached in every aspect of his life—even to the point of seeming at times a bit risqué and politically incorrect. He was often photographed enjoying a cigar. By all accounts he liked good Schnapps. Some might also call him an exhibitionist. At the studio, he rarely dressed in anything but the skimpiest shorts. Clara, by contrast, always wore a demure nurse's outfit. He was often seen running along the streets of New York in the dead of winter, naked, but for shoes and his trademark shorts.

He wore his whole life in plain view for all to see: prominent tattoos from his youth, a glass eye due to a boxing accident and, of course, his remarkable body, the surest proof that his method worked. "Although well past sixty," wrote one reviewer of his book, *Return to Life*, "Joseph H. Pilates owns a grand body that few men less than half his age ever attain. He has more suppleness than most college athletes." At the time of his death at age eighty-four, the *New York Times* described him as "a white-maned lion of a man, with steel blue eyes and mahogany skin . . . as limber in his eighties as a teenager."

His life was a testament to the power of the human spirit. Born sickly and asthmatic, he determined while still a boy to become not just healthy but a model of physical development. He succeeded beyond any reasonable expectation, eventually rehabilitating people from all walks of life.

Slowly, word of his methods grew. By the end of his life, the *New York Times* could report that his students and admirers included "actors, dancers, musicians, writers, and social figures, including Katherine Hepburn, Sir Laurence Olivier, Jose Ferrer, George Balanchine, Jerome Robbins, Roberta Peters, Maria Tallchief, Vera Zorina, and Gian Carlo Menotti." Famed modern dancer Ted Shawn called Joe's work "the finest system that I have ever known." As great as Joe's system was then for the rich and famous, its contemporary, the Pilates Method, has left an indelible mark in global citizens young and old, rich and poor, all seeking optimal health.

6

Chapter Six

Critique of the Human Condition

Joe was dismayed by the living conditions of modern industrial society. "Admittedly, it is rather difficult to gain ideal physical fitness under the handicap of daily breathing the soot-saturated air of our crowded and noisy cities. Even those of us who work in the city and are fortunate enough to live in the country must counteract the unnatural physical fatigue and mental strain experienced in our daily activities. Telephones, automobiles, and economic pressure all combine to create physical letdown and mental stress so great that today practically no home is entirely free from sufferers of some form of nervous tension." Joe's observations and conclusions of how pollution and stress hinder our ability to sustain physical fitness in body-mind are as true today for us, as they were for him.

Adding insult to injury, in Joe's opinion, standard medicine very often does not address the health needs of patients. After my own personal experiences with lengthy illness, I must concur. Western medicine's approach has its place and value in providing life saving interventions. But the day to day challenges to stay healthy in an ever changing global environment of pollutants and climate changes and conglomerate stresses of political unrest, a preventative, a more holistic approach to health, as Joe advised, would not only be advisable, but essential.

To Joe, it would seem that not much has changed for the improvement of a healthy body, mind, and spirit. "To one who has devoted the major portion of his life to the scientific study of the body and the prevention, rather than the cure, of disease," he wrote, "the misinformation I have so often listened to on the air, or read, borders closely on the criminal . . . because the acceptance of the theories thus advanced results in the actual shortening, instead of lengthening, of the lives of uncounted millions who fall for this bunk."

Joe's simple answer was his offer of the Pilates Method today; a system that "develops the body uniformly, corrects wrong postures, restores physical vitality, invigorates the mind, and elevates the spirit."

The practice of Pilates, he wrote, "is designed to give you suppleness, natural grace, and skill that will be unmistakably reflected in the way you walk, in the way you play, and in the way you work. You will develop muscular power with corresponding endurance, ability to perform arduous duties, to play strenuous games, to walk, run, or travel for long distances without undue body fatigue or mental strain. And this by no means is the end.

"By reawakening thousands and thousands of otherwise ordinarily dormant muscle cells, Contrology correspondingly reawakens thousands and thousands of dormant brain cells, thus activating new areas and stimulating further functioning of the mind. No wonder then that so many persons express such great surprise, following their initial experience with Contrology exercises, caused by their realization of the resulting sensation of 'uplift.' For the first time in many years their minds have been truly awakened."

Joe identified his work as Contrology: a 'control' that results in freedom, letting go of disempowering muscular and mental habits, patterns, and/or corresponding belief systems. There is freedom in releasing limiting habits (mind-body) and beliefs that no longer serve us. Here is where the 'space' to create something new within the mind-body happens.

The world was scarcely ready for Joe's message during his lifetime. But he left it anyway; he left it embedded in his Pilates Method. What had become evident to Joe was that health, "whole as one" was lost. At a time when the world faced a tipping point into the darker side of humanity, he wrote a letter to his clients as Germany invaded Poland—the opening sortie of World War II.

The lack of knowledge of general health on the people's part is largely responsible for world conditions today: responsible for combat, discouragement, crime, and premature death, because a healthy body—which most do not have—makes for a clean and healthy mind. It gives strength and decision of character and a directness of purpose, a love of refinement, purity, goodness, honor, justice, and morality. The mind, when housed within a healthy body, possesses a glorious sense of power. This world of ours is in turmoil and no one is positive of its outcome, and it is now more than ever before, more practicable and sensible, to be in a perfect state of health, both in body and in mind, in order to more successfully confront the problems continually arising.

—Joseph H. Pilates, September 1939 (Courtesy of The Pilates Center, Boulder, CO)

Joe's method strives to bring about a perceptual shift, a change in one's outlook from within, a sustainable resource of self-knowledge that can return one to a state of wholeness.

Now, more than four decades after his passing, Pilates is sweeping the globe. At the time of this writing, more than eleven million people with an excess of fourteen thousand teachers in the United States alone, and millions more in other countries, are flocking to Pilates classes at health clubs, YMCAs, gyms, and Pilates studios, and the numbers are growing by double-digit percentages every year.

Thanks to the vision and lifelong dedication of Joseph Pilates, his wife Clara, and a handful of original students, now known as the Pilates Elders, today, the Pilates Method is an idea whose time has come.

Part Two

The Pilates Approach to Total Health

The Pilates Approach to Total Health

"While the world is experiencing turbulent times . . . with wars, violence, and disease plaguing the earth, please realize that the apparent decay is precipitating vast evolutionary changes that will lead us to a far better reality. Knowledge, especially knowledge of self, is the key to our survival." —Biology of Belief, *Bruce Lipton, Ph.D., (Mountain of Love Productions, 2005)*

The power to change begins and ends with the individual. Self-knowledge is gained through expanded awareness and consciousness from within. That *inner* change in one's thoughts and beliefs elicits outer changes that can visibly be seen in one's life. These changes can be reflected in one or more life categories: work, relationships, recreation, and devotional practices. Today's landscape of the world—when what we do as individuals makes *a significant difference for the entire planet*—reminds us to live with reasonable balance and expanding awareness. The practice of Pilates instills both. Living with a deeper awareness and reasonable balance within these categories, one can begin to appreciate and integrate

Joe's statement that a healthy mind-body connection brings one *fully into life.*

Joe's method was initiated in self-awareness. Through the knowledge of his own body's limitations with disease, arose his need to create a healthier body. This need drove Joseph Pilates to discovery and that discovery fired his passions and his life's calling into his vision of health and vitality that would attract future generations of individuals seeking the same. Some individuals discovered—in their practice of the Pilates Method—paradigm shifts. For some the shifts were paramount in the physical body; for others, mental alertness became more acute, and still others, a *felt* sense of integration and wellness.

This is the real significance of Joseph Pilates' work: the practice of the Pilates Method as an adaptogen of holistic change in body, mind, and spirit. This, I believe, is the evolving work of Pilates today. Participating in healthy activities, like Pilates, supports us in recognizing and shifting old, repeating patterns that no longer serve us. Pilates creates the space in our mind-body connection for change to occur in how we move, think, and feel.

This book offers possibilities—steps to significant change—through the practice of the Pilates Method. *This* is where our contemporary world meets Joseph Pilates' world in a foundational understanding of how the mind-body connection, if adaptable, if willing, through *the work* reshapes, realigns, and redefines our lives in the physical, mental, emotional/social, and devotional aspects of our day to day activities. So, let the work begin. Step into your life!

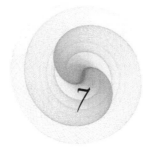

Chapter Seven

Change the Pattern

If you were to ask yourself what *controls* your health, your behavior, your preferences (likes/dislikes), or your happiness, would you know? I've asked myself those same questions over and over again. What if, as one cellular biologist and geneticist has suggested, *heredity* doesn't dictate destiny? What if *beliefs* influence our genes, too? Dr. Bruce H. Lipton, Ph.D., a cell biologist and author of *The Biology of Belief*, tells us that our cells are far more receptive to energy of thoughts and feelings than we ever imagined. "Traditional biology shows that cells communicate through chemical signals, like hormones. Recent research has discovered that cells communicate through electromagnetic energy signals. This is the same energy that makes up thought. In other words: beliefs control biology." *The Biology of Belief, Bruce Lipton, Ph.D., (Mountain of Love Productions, 2005)*

Perhaps our physiology creates pain and disease to give us feedback, to let us know we have an imbalanced perspective on life.

The word disease has been used for centuries. Its definition labels its victim and implies that your health is out of your control. It was in the early 1990s, shortly after my Pilates certification, that I noticed an alternative spelling, *dis-ease*. The hyphenated version of the word implies that an individual has ownership of his/her condition: *you are in a temporary state of discomfort over which you ultimately have control.*

"Disease is the result of a disruption of the spontaneous flow of nature's intelligence within our physiology," writes Virender Sodhi, MD (Ayurveda), ND, Director of the American School of Ayurvedic Sciences in Bellevue, Washington. (http://newyorkbodyscan.com/ayurvedic-medicine.html)

Our interpretation of what is or isn't a part of our reality has a profound impact on our perception of health and life.

The placebo effect would be a simple example of this. "Medicine is just beginning to use the mind-body connection for healing-defeating pain is a good example. By giving a placebo or dummy drug . . . patients will experience the same pain relief as if a real painkiller had been administered.

The pill itself is meaningless; the power that activates the placebo effect is the power of suggestion alone. This suggestion is then converted into the body's intention to cure itself. Therefore, why not bypass the deception of the sugar pill and go directly to the intention?" *Ageless Body, Timeless Mind*, Chopra, (Rider 1993)

At a purely physical level, Pilates is a great workout. At its most powerful, Pilates is an effective adaptogen to buffer the effect of the disruption we experience when not in the spontaneous flow of daily life. Left unattended, these disruptions can develop momentum, accelerating the numbing effects of stress, deadlines, and obligations. The practice of Pilates, from a whole body perspective, helps us recognize a symptom and respond accordingly.

This is in accordance with Joe's insight: "Practically all human ailments are directly traceable to wrong habits which can only be corrected through the immediate adoption of right (natural, normal) habits . . . only through the attainment of perfect balance of mind and body, can one appreciate what really constitutes normal health."

This 21st century interpretation of Pilates Contrology, my interpretation, and its inherent philosophy tells a story of how human beings can reach a fuller potential, in part, by adjusting their beliefs. *Knowledge is power and self-knowledge empowers the self to choose what one believes.* Joseph Pilates' work with the body was based in self-awareness: of breath, focus, intention, space, and movement toward vital health. Through this self-knowledge, Pilates can shift an individual's perception of possibility, thereby enhancing a life beyond expectation!

Chapter Eight

Experiencing "It"

During my years of teaching Pilates to clients and assisting Wendy LeBlanc-Arbuckle in training future teachers through the Core Connections® Pilates Certification program at The Pilates Center of Austin (PCA), I have seen passion drive people of all ages, abilities, and former life tracks to leave established professions in order to become Pilates teachers. Why? I believe it has something to do with what begins to shift for them personally.

Some of the teacher trainees felt such a strong desire toward Pilates as a lifestyle of greater awareness and service toward others that they left careers that they'd fully invested in for three decades, all highly educated in either industry or academia.

They felt the effect of Pilates practice on their own bodies—a unified expression of mind-body—so *inspired* was their heart's desire, their visions, their joy of celebration in a new found lifestyle—that they wanted to share this expanded life experience with others.

Here is an example of one of those individuals.

Brenda has been doing Pilates for about nine years. During most of that time she was a professional interior designer, but two years ago she changed careers and became a Pilates instructor. At the time of this writing, she is forty-three years old. I asked Brenda what had motivated her to try Pilates in the first place.

"I was running long distances, and I was starting to feel some achiness in my knees and hips," she told me. "I love to run, and I thought . . . *I don't want to end up where I can't do this. Am I doing something wrong that I can correct, just body mechanics?* So I looked in the phone book and found a Pilates teacher. She sold me on it, so I went in. I remember attending my first session, and I remember leaving there feeling taller, lighter, energized . . . the whole thing."

Brenda stands five foot two. "After I'd done Pilates for about a year," she says, "I was an inch taller, which is very cool. I need that inch."

Before long, she became passionate about doing Pilates. "I started doing one session a week, and then it grew to two, then three. It was something that I made sure I had time for. I couldn't imagine any reason that I would miss it. I would go no matter what. As I'm doing it, I'm thinking: *Other people should know about this.* I mean, I felt so good, and I was running my best ever. I had no pain at all. People need to hear about this."

I have witnessed Brenda's kind of enthusiasm in countless Pilates clients and practitioners. The awareness we develop as teachers stems from the inquiry: *How has Pilates served me?* Many of us have come to Pilates from the pain and disability of injury. Injury is not limited to the physical. Injury occurs from impact of relationships, environment, and interference of our daily routines.

Numerous conversations with colleagues and clients here and abroad established my understanding of the benefits of Pilates as common ground to all who do the work:

> *As Pilates teachers—because we first had to experience 'it' in our bodies, and now wish to transfer that knowledge to others—we recognize that the expression of ourselves* now *is not the same as when we started* then. *Since then, we have been attempting to explain this experience that goes beyond learning and teaching mere physical exercise.*

I believe it is this elusive nuance, coming from an unconscious place in our psyche or soul, which drives us to this dedication. So many of those who teach this method—especially teaching Pilates to those recovering from accidents or injuries—teach from a place of *compassion.* Their approach to the work is from a position of service *to uplift the human condition from suffering.*

In fact, according to Wayne Dyer, research studies have proven the positive effect of compassion on the immune system and on the increased production of serotonin in the brain. "Research has shown that a simple act of kindness directed toward another improves the functioning of the immune system and stimulates the production of serotonin in both the recipient of the kindness and the person extending the kindness. Even more amazing is that persons observing the act of kindness have similar beneficial results. Imagine this! Kindness extended, received, or observed beneficially impacts the physical health and feelings of everyone involved!"

It's not hard to understand why Pilates' popularity has exploded in recent years. Individuals—to their astonishment—discover they can become more of who they intended to be, beyond the physical result of exercise. They find that living life itself is grander than what they had previously known. You find yourself saying 'Yes!' to life.

Again, I asked Brenda what it was about the practice of Pilates that most influenced her to change her career. "It was a gradual thing," she told me. "When I started doing Pilates, I would leave the studio feeling so good, feeling that there was so much more to life than what I was doing, so much more purpose. I think, for me, connecting the mind to the body was huge. It just opened up everything else within my world."

I asked her what she finds most gratifying about helping others do Pilates.

"When they tell me that they no longer have pain in their bodies," she said. "When they see a difference, and feel different, that's the whole goal."

The reduction of symptoms—primarily pain or restricted motion—is among the most often reported outcomes of Pilates practice. Almost always, though, the benefits of Pilates involve more than just the body.

"I see not only the changes that the body has made," Brenda told me, "but the changes that the mind makes right along with it. David is a perfect example." When Brenda first saw David as a client, he was sixty-five years old and carrying two hundred and eighty pounds on his six-foot-four-inch frame. "He came in absolutely the most de-conditioned client I had," Brenda recalls. "He had done nothing physically for a long time. Doctors had told him he needed to do something, but they hadn't guided him on what to do. I train his wife, and she really wanted him to try Pilates, so he came in. We started out just doing the very basics. All the basic stuff was very hard for him."

As it turned out, Pilates gave David the means to transform his life. Since starting with Brenda, he has lost thirty pounds, but that was only the beginning of his changes. "He has goals in his mind," Brenda said. "He's so excited to try something new. He wants to start doing karate. Pilates has just given him a zest for life."

Zest for life—the very thing that Joseph Pilates promised would return to anyone who practices Contrology. In David's case, this also involved relief of great pain in his lower back as he regained his suppleness and range of motion. "He told me he was in pain all the time," Brenda said. "Just carrying around that much weight is hard on the spine. Starting out, after probably a couple of months, he tried a Pilates exercise called long stretch. He did one, and he went down to his knees and said it was too hard. He can now do the entire Long Stretch Series in perfect form. This is progress!"

The change in David is obvious to those around him. Brenda recalls that when she first met him he seemed "very downtrodden, very tired. Now he stands tall, and his eyes sparkle." Brenda concludes: "Pilates changes your outlook on things, not only on yourself and your own body, but on how you view the world."

Joe said, "Correct the habit." (Change the pattern.) This is the richer harvest you reap from Pilates. You are then shifting your patterns of how you move in the world. Cooperation and compassion within ourselves and in how we relate to others becomes the rule, rather than the exception.

Here again the Pilates Method ushers us into a more authentic self, reversing the adverse effects of base consciousness into a more sustainable wisdom. As Mary Bowen, a first-generation Pilates instructor who blends Jungian analysis with Pilates, says about the deeper nature of Joseph Pilates' work: "Joe meant to inform every moving moment in your life. He wanted to change the world."

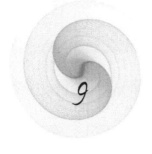

Chapter Nine

Three Key Themes

The word *health* is derived from the Greek root *holos* or 'whole.' Healing, as I learned through Pilates, is something greater than the total sum of its respective parts. This wholeness implies complete unification as one body, mind, and spirit.

Joe Pilates wrote: "Contrology is complete coordination of body, mind, and spirit. Through Contrology you first purposefully acquire complete control of your own body and then through proper repetition of its exercises you gradually and progressively acquire that natural rhythm and coordination associated with all your subconscious activities." *Return to Life Through Contrology,* (1945)

Brenda realized this after doing Pilates for only a short time. As she says, "It just opened up everything else within my world. I had never done an exercise where the mind was so present."

What opened up for me personally was a *world of possibilities*. There was a definite correlation between the practice of Pilates and the expanded awareness of clients; not just the changes taking place within their own bodies, but changes in how they perceived themselves in their relationships, work, etc. My ongoing Pilates training fed this notion that the Pilates Method is a truly powerful path to "the acquirement and enjoyment of physical well-being, mental calm, and spiritual peace." *Return to Life Through Contrology*, (1945)

Interpreted through Joe's written work, Pilates addresses each of these bodies, *well being, mental calm, and spiritual peace,* giving rise to a *renewed felt sense* of *self.* All are favorable results in body, mind, and spirit.

Pilates teachers I've interviewed have observed time and time again in working with clients that they consistently achieve these three key themes:

- OUTCOMES: The reduction of symptoms—*well being*

- PERCEPTIONS: Enhanced mental clarity—*mental calm*

- LIVING LIFE FULLY: A feeling of lightness—*spiritual peace*

Let's take a closer look at these themes and their role in the Pilates path to total health.

Well Being The idea of reducing symptoms is not usually associated with the kind of physical exercise one finds at a gym or fitness center. In fact, without proper preparedness or supervision, symptoms may *start* during intense exercise like weight training or competitive sports—symptoms such as lasting soreness in the spine, knees, shoulders, or various kinds of painful muscle strain. Just as often, however, such symptoms result from de-conditioning: the gradual degradation of overall fitness so commonly associated with high-stress, low-activity lifestyles, *or simply being unaware of what would feel different from that. Pilates holds the space for possibility.* Pilates, under proper supervision, invariably *reduces* symptoms, often to the surprise and huge relief of the client who may have lived with debilitating pain for years, resigned to the belief that pain was permanent and inescapable. Transformation of symptoms becomes approachable and attainable.

When a person lives with chronic pain, Western medicine typically takes one of two approaches: pharmaceutical pain management or surgery. Neither of these healing modalities is guaranteed to end a patient's pain or bring them to full recovery. While these approaches may temporarily lessen the symptoms while engaged in a lengthy recovery, there are potential side effects in either scenario.

By contrast, Pilates, when properly taught and practiced, more often than not, results in reduced pain and improved range of motion, usually in a matter of weeks or at most, a few months, so that drugs or invasive procedures may not be needed. These outcomes are accompanied by a gradual but inevitable increase in strength, suppleness, energy level, and overall sense of well-being and conditioning. This all comes down to a matter of *creating space in the body* through awareness.

Stephanie, a longtime Pilates enthusiast, author, and owner of a publishing company devoted to wellness materials, has this observation about self-awareness through her Pilates practice:

> "Awareness is a multi-level system which Pilates activates and unifies. For example, having to release my sternum made me aware that I was rigidly guarding my heart. It was palpable how fear and anxiety were constricting my heart space. Holding my breath was how I held my sternum in an armoring position. I then noticed that this posture created tension between my shoulder blades as well as in the mid-back. Today, this connection between an emotional state of fear and anxiety, and a physical state of tension and pain, *is now under my own control.* And when I adjust the physical state by tuning in, by anchoring my feet and breathing myself into a lifted posture, I move from emotional/physical tension and pain to joy and freedom of movement."

This experience of awareness, creating a window of opportunity to see herself clearly and distinguish needs related to her well being, is not unique to Stephanie. Pilates reawakens an innate knowledge, an inner propriety, which for all intents and purposes is a misplaced blueprint to health. Like a lost artifact that has always been there, once found, it can be dusted off, reassembled if broken, and put to its useful purpose.

Mental Calm describes a shift that occurs in a Pilates training session in your ability to think clearly and focus. A veil or fog lifts from your mind and any sluggish processing disappears. Pilates applies a method of focus that employs a quality of attention, expressed through a wide assortment of highly specific movements performed on a mat or on the unique Pilates equipment. These movements do not require interminable repetitions wherein the mind wanders where it will, but rather engages a unique mix of breath, balance, and heightened awareness that elicits power—a quality of attention unlike anything you may have put your mind to.

An experienced Pilates practitioner knows you can't force your way through exercises to get the result you are looking for—there is thoughtful consideration to do them in your best interest and achieve a greater outcome—a unification of body, mind, and spirit, 'that which supports the significance of life itself.' *Power vs. Force*, David R. Hawkins, (Hay House, 2002)

This is what Brenda found so eye-opening about her initial Pilates sessions: the presence of *mind* in every moment of the experience. "I had never done an exercise where the mind was so present, where I was using my brain as much as I was using my muscles," she said.

Pilates intentionally demands that every client use his/her mind, not only to perform a movement successfully, but also to discern how that movement is affecting the body. In this way, clients soon become true architects of the space inside their bodies; and in so doing, they enhance their own mind-body connection to a degree that many find startling and exhilarating. I recall one of my clients saying that she loved Pilates because "It's the hardest thing I've ever done!"

What she is referring to is not only the exercise, but also the awareness and mental effort needed to execute the exercise. This is what is meant by *working out from within*.

As we practice Pilates—beyond the movement—we are informing our parts, through thought, *into a* body *of knowledge, and arrive at a unified whole,* **within** *where spirit resides. There is the possibility that through the acquired movements of Pilates, we <u>feel</u> clearer, we <u>think</u> clearer, and <u>our intention in the world is clearer</u>.* We transform the quality of our life through our influence on the perception of the world around us.

Body (embodiment)	symptoms	BODY
Thought (perception)	mental clarity	MIND
Form (space)	passion / purpose lightness	SPIRIT

Spiritual Peace The spiritual component of Pilates is perhaps best reflected in a shift in perspective of life, redefining purpose and passion, and a newfound sense of lightness that clients bring to the activities of daily living. This shift is, in common Pilates parlance, called a change in *altitude*—a sense of higher vibration, higher functioning, finer attunement with the essence of one's own being—*a lightness*.

Joy or happiness, an essential ingredient of health, is an intended outcome of the regular practice of Pilates. Joe once said, "The whole world should do my exercises. They'd be happier." (Pilate Method Alliance, The 100's Newsletter)

Once an individual chooses to separate from conditioned patterns and constructs, she begins to live in a childlike state of freedom, a kind of bliss that reminds you that you are lighter than the weightiness of the external world.

Stephanie describes her newfound sense of freedom: "The joy that suddenly shows up is a feeling very much like I experience when swimming, or when I did gymnastics as a child. It needs no reason to be there—it just flows in, filling the space created by the Pilates experience. I think it comes from the fact that becoming aware of the space inside myself, as a human body, exploring what is possible, is the ultimate playfulness. Unlike the happiness I feel momentarily when I buy a great pair of shoes, this joy seems to spring from the exhilarating sense of freedom that leaps into my heart when I've broken free of some internal limitation."

The resulting spiritual peace embodies the essence of Joe's work, a _uniquely coordinated trinity of balance_; body, mind, and spirit that has its affect as a reduction of symptoms, increased mental clarity, and a return to passion and purpose in life. This spiritual enhancement is what clients take home with them from their Pilates practice; what they carry with them out into today's world.

10

Chapter Ten

Moving Beyond Limitations

Inevitably, we find ourselves in some sort of head on collision with what we didn't expect our life path to encounter. Pilates offers a way through when life's challenges seem insurmountable. Laura's experience is a powerful testimony to what is possible for all those who seem to think they cannot overcome their perceived limitations. For Laura the challenges of daily living after an auto accident were staggering. We met as client and teacher after her eight years from the onset of that collision, culminating into a history of baffling symptoms that left her bound to an indeterminate future of the same. For anyone having such diminished energy from inactivity, it can feel like a slow decline into an abyss, a way out of what seems impossible.

Here is a list of some things that Pilates can impact and which most of us have available in our lives. *Imagine if these daily functions were unavailable, or at best elusive in your life!?*

This was the case in Laura's life before Pilates.

What wasn't possible or was painful:

- Brushing teeth

- Unloading a washer

- Fixing hair

- Talking on a phone

- Keyboarding

- Sleeping

- Sitting

- Walking

What is possible now and not as painful:

All of the above, along with:

- Driving

- Traveling in cars, planes, buses

- Writing

- Ironing

- Some household chores

- Bicycling

- Dog training

- Needlework

- Muscle coordination

For Laura, discovery—from what seemed impossible—has been an ongoing process. She says, "It is linked congruently with self-knowledge. Along the way I would discover things—such as if my neck muscles would relax, the pain in my hand would decrease. The discoveries of how the body, as a whole, is affected by limitations, even in the smaller parts of the body (hand or foot), opened my awareness to greater possibilities. My attention to that end revealed an effort with ease that wasn't happenstance, but congruent with my new found thoughts. With Pilates, the most interesting discovery is how different parts of the body are affected positively to work in harmony with other parts of the body. This reconnection of relationships within me is something I haven't experienced in eight years!"

Pilates can be served up in a fashion that fits your lifestyle, meeting you where you are, whether in rehabilitation with an injury or preparing for the Olympics. Pilates is unique in that it addresses the individual as a whole, whether a professional dancer, office worker, homemaker, engineer, athlete, or retired senior citizen, Pilates can create the same experience of health from within.

The Pilates Method is more than addressing body parts and pieces. It is an exploration and discovery of self through the mind-body connection. The outcome of which is a shift in one's identity: moment by moment, or developmentally, students notice the gradual and constant improvement of patterns that no longer serve their bodies, minds, or spirits. A reasonable balance returns.

In 2004, I listened to a lecture by a colleague and friend, Brent Anderson, P.T., President and Co-founder of Polestar Pilates, an international teacher training organization. As one who has evolved Joe's original work into rehabilitation techniques that are now employed by Polestar Pilates rehabilitation specialists worldwide, Brent posed this profound challenge to his diverse audience: "It comes down to *a belief* model that tends to be the greatest predictor of somebody getting better or not. If *this* is the biggest predictor of outcome, how does Pilates affect belief model?" His astute audience worked through the basic tenets of Joe Pilates' philosophy, observing the importance of self-control and perception in healing oneself and discerned the following:

- Understand *breath* as metaphor, the awareness of self, and respiration as science, the physiology of breathing.

- Bring movement back to *function*.

- Create *self-control* in perception.

- Heighten *awareness*.

- *Empower* people to be involved with their health.

Brent concluded that when people "see that they have control over certain parts of their lives," it decreases their perception of pain.

Control

There is no such 'thing' as too old to come into this sense of being; this path to healing. A great initiative for the Pilates client is the awesome teacher who ushers you into and holds this much needed attentive space for you to rediscover a deeper sense of fitness and health. This is a distinctive quality in the relationship between the Pilates teacher and student. Many students are taking lifelong lessons, affirming that the Pilates Method is a lifestyle choice for health and fitness. To realize the transformational powers of Pilates, both teacher and student must be coming from the possibility that Pilates is transformational, not just *doing* exercises.

According to Deepak Chopra, "Every experience comes to us in one of four ways: a feeling, a thought, an action, or simply a sense of being. When an experience is so powerful that it motivates people to change the whole pattern of their lives, this is called an epiphany." *The Book of Secrets: Unlocking the Hidden Dimensions of Your Life,* (Random House Audio, 2004)

As humankind is able to upgrade its expansion of awareness and consciousness, the consciousness of health is a natural next step. Those actively practicing and teaching Pilates as a venue for health can open a space that creates the possibility that Pilates can reach out globally and bring the practice of the Pilates Method to any individual or any community. Joseph Pilates brought *his concept* to the internment camps in England in World War I, (bringing stamina, strength, flexibility, and health to those prisoners who practiced his method with him, surviving the harshest of conditions enabling them to walk out of the camps.) It is here that the Pilates legacy of Joe is renewed, lives, and breathes with possibilities, and personifies Joseph Pilates' desire to change the world.

The following chart considers this power of individual consciousness:

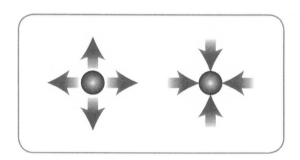

Each one of these dots has a certain quality of existence on this page. Which looks restricted and bounded? Which appears to have a global reference to itself? Which has a local reference to itself? The arrows indicate applied force or applied power. In which direction would that be? Which quality of existence would you like to express? Which do you think Pilates subscribes to? This is what can happen when Pilates is in your body and your life.

Having initially described the powerful mind, body, and spirit connection of Pilates, we now look more specifically at the basic principles of Contrology and how they work to provide the path to total health that Joe envisioned and that lives on through Pilates instruction today.

Part Three

The Six Principles
of Pilates

The Six Principles of Pilates

"These ideas or concepts will drive your experience. Through these steps you can begin to adjust to a different perspective . . . as you transition toward that of a universal human being." —Lisette Larkins

Imagine Joseph Pilates pacing the floor of his New York studio, barking out instructions to his students in a thick German accent: "You must **concentrate** to get **control** of your **center!** **Flowing movement** will come with the **precision** of your **breath!**"

Six principles—concentration, control, centering, flowing movement, precision, and breathing—were extrapolated by Phillip Friedman and Gail Eisen in *The Pilates Method of Physical and Mental Conditioning*, (Doubleday, 1980) as their interpretation from Pilates' original philosophy as expounded in his *Return to Life Through Contrology* (1945). As a start point for developing our understanding of what is possible when evoking the aforementioned six principles, each will be preempted by a direct reference from Friedman and Eisen's interpretation. As you read, consider that language evolves through time, as do the words to convey any idea. Since then, an array of descriptive synonyms have been added to the mix to illuminate the thoughts originally expressed with relative terms like; *core strength, attentive relaxation, whole body movement, alignment, and integration.* Rather than a description like: determinant strength of your muscles corresponding to body image as your Pilates experience; perhaps, a deeper awareness like, *how well your mind and body coordinate for any movement which enhances your life experience.*

Here we explore these words, old and new, and hopefully come to an understanding of how Pilates can be a journey through—and an experience of—what is possible in renewing one's life. These original six words lend themselves as principles and give clarity to the facets of Joe's method, not only an approach to understanding how to do it, but ultimately recognizing *whole body health. And* these original six classical principles—now doctrine in the eyes of many contemporary practitioners, are the touchstones which distinguish Joe's work in many learning environments, from the small-town gym to the most elite Pilates studios and cutting-edge physical therapy clinics around the world.

In *Return to Life Through Contrology,* Joe's philosophical concepts preceded a compilation of thirty-four exercises at the end of the book, *implying that one must first understand the principles and philosophy before pursuing the exercises. With the principles understood—an essential element of embodiment*—the body is primed to assimilate the information contained in each exercise, information that will gradually be translated into intelligence for the 'thousands of dormant cells' that govern our being. This awakening process—which literally occurs at the cellular level, the aforementioned cells now known to be in the trillions (the study of which today is referenced as *new edge science*)—is what Joe meant by a "return to life." The uniqueness in a Pilates movement is that your attention on yourself is global, not on separate parts and pieces, and you are **expanding** your awareness physically and mentally.

The concept that one can renew health and return to life implies that, for many people, the 'normal' state is not fully alive. Contrology therefore poses a profound challenge to the status quo. In our 'normal' state, we are only partially awake, only partly aware of our innate capabilities and potential. Through the movements of Pilates—not just a series of exercises, but exercise governed by six principles, which when integrated, define a concrete, practical path to a life that is fully awake, aware, and able to express its innate potential—we find ourselves becoming more fully who we truly are; we evolve our current nature to something fuller, more alive.

Let's take a closer look at these six principles, one by one, not only as it was postulated that Joe embodied them in his teaching, but also as we have come to understand and experience them at the dawn of the 21st century.

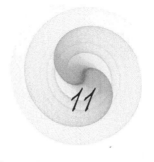

Chapter Eleven

Breathing

Though some discussions of the six principles place breathing last, it is so fundamental to Pilates in theory and practice that I prefer to place it first. If you aren't breathing, you aren't alive. Movement animates life and breath eliminates fatigue.

"For the blood to do its work properly, it has to be charged with oxygen and purged of waste gases, and that means proper breathing." *The Pilates Method of Physical and Mental Conditioning*, Phillip Friedman and Gail Eisen, (Doubleday and Company, 1980)

To this end—*full and thorough inhalation and exhalation are a part of every Pilates exercise.* Pilates spoke of complete exhalation as the key to full inhalation. "Squeeze out the lungs as you would wring a wet towel dry," he is reputed to have said. Pilates breathing brings insight to qualities of attention like concentration, control, and precision which create a pathway to find a natural breath. Today, allowing the body to breathe in a conducive manner, practitioners assert, not only oxygenates the muscles, but also reduces tension in the upper neck and shoulders. Pilates breathing is described as a posterior lateral breathing, meaning that the student/client can explore inhaling naturally by leading the breath toward the back and sides of his or her rib cage. The exhale would be described as sensing a drop and deepening of the abdomen while noting the engagement of deep abdominal muscles, maintaining this engagement without tension as the next inhale begins. Pilates attempts to properly coordinate this breathing practice with movement, including breathing instructions with every exercise. Joseph Pilates stated, "Even if you follow no other instructions, learn to breathe correctly." Better breath means more energy, which means a better quality of life.

Do not forget

Years ago a doctor referred a twelve-year-old patient to me who was afflicted with cerebral palsy. This was not your typical person seeking an exercise program, but a young boy shaking uncontrollably when he walked and stuttering when he spoke. I remember the look on the faces of my receptionist and a fellow teacher in the room when this boy came in. You could have heard a pin drop. All eyes were on me, begging the question: *What in the world are you going to do here?* I didn't know. Frankly, I was nervous, and felt humbled in this boy's presence.

"How can I help you today?" I asked him.

The boy stuttered back, "My doctor thinks this can help my condition."

"What is it about your condition you need help with?"

The boy replied, "I don't have much control of myself."

My eyes filled up with tears, and I swallowed hard. "Well, why don't I make you comfortable, and we can start with breathing."

A couple of weeks later a postcard showed up in the mail. It was hand written with obvious effort. It read: *"dear Gary, thank you for teaching me how to breathe it helps me manage myself better when i am having a bad day."* Though I did not see this client again, I knew that my simple instruction in helping him be more comfortable with his breathing had been for him life-changing.

Pilates exercises were designed to help us breathe better, whether lying on a mat or on the equipment. The act of breathing prescribed by Joe is not the way you have breathed all your life. But, then, you probably didn't have asthma as he did, and in his time, there wasn't an atomizer to counteract the narrowing of the lungs' air passageways. Back then, Joe's life depended on learning to breathe as fully and efficiently as possible. He had to become aware of his breathing, and discovered that to get an adequate inhalation into your lungs you must have a complete and thorough exhalation, now known as the 'Pilates breath.'

"Breathing is the first act of life and the last. To breathe correctly you must completely *exhale* and inhale, always trying very hard to squeeze every atom of impure air from your lungs," he wrote. He further explains, "To properly deflate the lungs is an art in itself . . . it is seldom, if ever, properly taught . . . by one who understands what it really is all about."

[handwritten: Exhale completely, like Feldenkrass. pause. Let inhalation happen naturally,]

[handwritten margin: let breath inspire you]

Joe's awareness on how to exhale gives rise to inhalation arriving fully into the deepest and most healthful part of your lungs, the lower lobes. This breath gave him back his health, renewed his life, and inspired him to create ingenious equipment and movements to sustain a better life for others! This style of breathing is the path to mastery for his prescribed exercises.

Viewing Pilates through a 21st century lens, I have come to realize that each of Joseph Pilates' six principles has an important metaphysical correlate, and that *a particular quality of mind (thought) connects to the action of the body (embodiment).* (Each of these metaphysical correlates will be described in the following chapters.) With respect to breathing:

The metaphysical correlate to breathing is awareness of self, and the connecting quality is attention.

The breath represents awareness, spirit, the life-force—when we bring our attention to it.

In order to help you track your breath, just follow along. Lying on your back with knees bent and a small pillow under your head, put your hands on your stomach and notice that when your stomach isn't rising on your inhalation you have controlled your breath to move into your lungs more deeply. Or, put your hands along the sides of your ribcage. Notice you are filling your ribcage, its sides and back, with air in place of noticing your belly rising. Visualize this act of breathing as you do it. If appropriate for you, you can add this visualization whenever you need to find that quiet place within yourself. *"Breath in through your nose, down your throat, and let it warm your heart."*

Let this phrase help track your breath. Do this lying down on your bed at the beginning or end of your day. Get comfortable and put a couple of pillows under your knees. Feel the release of the tension you hold. Feel how your exhalation can be greater than you've previously experienced, and how, upon release, the muscles around your spine relax. Notice that the exhalation allows your bones to release and connect onto the surface you are lying on. This newfound breath pattern may suggest a meditative state that whispers *"Go deeper on your exhalation."* This is a state of attentive relaxation

In our society, breathing is largely taken for granted. It is through attention and awareness of self through the breath that we tap into our relationship with everything: our connectedness, our purpose, and our *full attentive presence of self.*

Now you're ready to focus your mind on what is at hand. Thus we arrive at the second principle, Concentration.

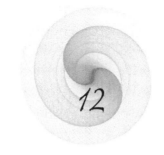

Chapter Twelve

Concentration

Concentration is focused attention, immersion, or absorption in mental effort. This is the necessary quality of *attention*—being fully present *in the moment*—in a Pilates session. Focused attention brings with it power. The quality of attention you bring has with it greater gains that aren't always obvious.

"You must concentrate on what you are doing. All of the time. And you must concentrate on your entire body." *The Pilates Method of Physical and Mental Conditioning*, Philip Friedman and Gail Eisen, (Doubleday and Company, 1980)

As Joe advised: "Concentrate on the correct movements EACH TIME YOU EXERCISE, lest you do them improperly and thus lose all the vital benefits of their value. Correctly executed and mastered to the point of subconscious reaction, these exercises will reflect grace and balance in your routine activities."

His emphasis on "each time you exercise" suggests *cohesiveness or a quality of attention that makes a difference.*

He also emphasized the *"vital benefits of their value."* That statement implies you don't have the benefits of Pilates until you pay attention to the quality of what you are doing. *Subconscious attainment is the goal of this attentiveness.* Pilates is not an event outside yourself. The event is within you.

Listening to neuroscientist Candace Pert, Ph.D., I realized an important correlation to Pilates, "The word 'mind' really means 'to pay attention to.' Developing the ability to choose what we want to pay attention to is a mark of evolutionary advancement." We as a species are continually evolving. Our ability to stay focused in the moment—or an hour Pilates session—matters.

Further, as the Taylor sisters' explain in *The Everything Pilates Book,* concentration and awareness go hand in hand: "Concentration and awareness are like the micro-focus and the macro-focus functions of a single lens. You need to be able to both concentrate on the specifics and be aware of the whole. Awareness makes you 'present' in every Pilates movement and exercise. In the course of any series of Pilates movements, your body is in a continual state of evolution."

Thus concentration has an expanded meaning in twenty-first-century vernacular . . . awareness. Following is a diagram of how you can evolve from concentration to awareness, and eventually to rediscovering one's passion.

Concentration ⟶ Awareness ⟶ Consciousness ⟶ Self-Realization ⟶ Spirit

A particularly vivid example of such personal evolution is told by Sean, a high school student and track athlete, who was in chronic pain from a hiking injury that interfered with his sport and his life. Facing knee pain, hamstring tightness, and a pulled transverse abdominis—the deepest, if not the most serious, abrasion of stomach muscles, he felt anguished at the thought of not being in control of his destiny.

"I knew all of these problems were connected, but I was frustrated because I had no way of changing the source they stemmed from—or even, at that time, knowing what that source was. I was at the mercy of health professionals, who gave me temporary relief and mixed advice. My abdominal injury made most movement painful, and I had to put most physical activity on hiatus.

Following is his declaration of how he perceives himself, and the world around him, after less than one year of Pilates:

> "Ultimately, what turned my grief into relief was a new *awareness* of myself. Fast forwarding a little less than one year, since Pilates, I am doing both of the movements that had caused injury in the past—running down the side of a mountain after summiting it—with loose hamstrings. I felt great satisfaction, relief, and confidence with every pain-free, efficient step I took."

> "Eventually, it seems so simple it's ludicrous: in order to increase awareness of our minds, hearts . . . and spirituality, we must increase awareness of

our bodies, every second of the day. The concept is indeed very simple: understanding, controlling, and consciously moving the body at all times."

Taking a closer look at what Sean is alluding to and how an epiphany like this could occur in one's perception, we are reminded of the discussion in Part Two about mind, body, and spirit connection resulting in *well being, mental calm, and spiritual peace.* These three factors give rise to a *renewed felt sense* of *self.* Sean echoes this idea:

> "There are few lucky people who will discover the correct way to live. Few who will realize the inherent happiness and enlightenment that manifests as human consciousness, and few who will find a teacher to help bring them to said realization. But those few must learn how to move correctly, how to be still correctly—from the body to the mind, and inevitably to the elusive spirit that is one with both movement—body—and mind."

I also had a personal experience with awareness during a Beginner/Intermediate session at The Pilates Center teacher training program in Boulder. I was in a group of prospective Pilates teachers using the Pilates apparatus known as the Reformer. Romana Kryzanowska, a 1st Generation Pilates Teacher, was teaching us. I was struggling with previous hamstring injuries, and when we got to Splits, I expressed my concern. Her emphatic response was, "You are healed!" I realized then that I was healed! Considering the foundation work that I had just performed, it was just a matter of me creating a perceptual shift into doing the Splits. And I did!

If, instead of focusing on what I was presently doing, I had put my mental energy into how it's always been or how it might be in the future, I would never have been able to do splits on the reformer. This poses a question, how good are we at holding our power in the moment or being here now? Sometimes, we tend to define our self by our worst moment rather than noticing that knowing our limitations is progress toward overcoming them.

You may not have chosen what happened *to you*—but you can choose what you do with it.

To make this choice requires you enter the presence of mind that brings you into the "now." Much of what we do in life puts our focus and attention outside ourselves. All the pressures and concerns from the dictates outside ourselves limit our expression of what truly is.

The metaphysical correlate to concentration is present moment awareness, and the connecting quality is being in the now.

The present is the most powerful time/place in a person's life, as there is possibility for action and change. Having a flash of insight, or an epiphany, is an "unspoken" benefit of Pilates a day, week, or month after a session.

This presence of mind, being here now, stems from an ancient revelation. In his book, *Power, Freedom, and Grace,* Deepak Chopra shares with us his Indian-Vedic tradition:

"Going back within myself, I create again and again. I create the mind, I create the body, I create perceptions, I create the universe. I create all things that I call reality."

This ancient wisdom of "going back within myself" is echoed by Wendy LeBlanc-Arbuckle, who says that the possibility of Pilates can be a continuum for looking deeply within our felt sense, being willing to not judge, inspiring us to embody ourselves and celebrate a truly new moment. At The Pilates Center of Austin we called it "living life with passion, purpose, and vitality." Just as Joseph Pilates speaks of Contrology as a "return to life."

Once we find this present moment awareness, that leads us to the next principle, control.

Chapter Thirteen

Control

The essence of Contrology is found in its root: control. While practicing Pilates, each exercise must be executed with control in order to reap the benefits and prevent injury. By taking control of your mind, muscles, and bones through movement, you take control of your body and your health.

"Nothing about the Pilates Method is haphazard. The reason you need to concentrate so thoroughly is so you can be in control of every aspect of every movement." *The Pilates Method of Physical and Mental Conditioning*, Philip Friedman and Gail Eisen, (Doubleday and Company, 1980)

This idea of 'control '—that the only thing we can control is ourselves—results in freedom, letting go of disempowering muscular habits or patterns and corresponding belief systems. Letting go of limiting belief systems asks us to re-discover potential and relinquish doubt. Robert Collier (1885–1950), a philosopher of Joseph Pilates' era, said, "All power is from within and is therefore under our own control."

This is John's story of how, by choosing to be open to what is possible, gained control of his life through Pilates. John was involved in a motorcycle accident that left him with a serious limp and chronic pain. At six-foot-four and two hundred eighty pounds, he was de-conditioned due to multiple fractures in his right femur that had shortened his leg. A high school teacher, he normally spent most of his working day on his feet. By age fifty-eight, when John came to me for help, his pain was becoming too much to bear. "If it hadn't been for Pilates," John told me later, "I think last year I would have retired at the end of the year, because I was in that much pain. But what we did last year from about September through April really allowed me to say that maybe I can go another year. And I did."

John discovered that regaining control of his life started with taking control of his movement patterns. "Pilates got me in the habit, the routine, of stretching every morning, getting up and doing stretching exercises," he says. "It just set the tone for the whole day." As a result of taking control of his movements, after relearning how to stretch from an *anchored position of stability*, he regained flexibility and the ability to walk without a limp. The pain in his hips and lower back was greatly reduced, and he recovered mobility that had been lost. "I was able to do all kinds of things at school," he told me, "lift and bend and stretch and carry things that I wasn't able to do before."

Pilates not only gave John the opportunity to continue in his teaching job, but it also allowed him to return to other activities he loved, including kayaking and hiking in the mountains. For John, getting control of the basic ability to walk correctly and minimize pain meant a significant 'return to life.'

Our lack of vision or lack of understanding can sometimes hinder our true nature to self-heal and would keep us limited in a cycle of pain.

Through our unawareness we are left without conscious choice—functioning with parts and not the whole of who we are. With Pilates, John's way of thinking changed. John opened up to uncharted possibility.

"I used to hesitate to do a lot of things because of the effort it took to get going," he says. "When you're able to walk naturally and normally, it certainly increases the quality of life—not only what you're able to do but what you're interested in doing."

The metaphysical correlate to control is conscious choice, and the connecting quality is self-knowledge.

This newfound sense of control is a form of self-knowledge. Pilates teaches us that by consciously choosing to take control, we can release self-limiting beliefs that have kept us locked in painful, unworkable life patterns. What can make something unworkable is our inexperience. We are not bound by circumstances, but only by our willingness to let circumstances control us. Circumstances change when we open up, physically and mentally, to the possibilities.

Pilates is not a quick-fix fitness program. It is a lifelong undertaking in developing self-knowledge. Perhaps the most famous dictum in all of Greek philosophy is: 'Know thyself.'

Historians tell us that these words were inscribed in gold over the entrance to the temple of Apollo at Delphi. To the ancient Greeks—and to Joseph Pilates—*know thy self* begins with knowing your body.

The greatest gift you will receive from Pilates is that you will get to know yourself. Pilates meets you at the level where you find yourself right now. You progress by building on what you are learning, enhancing self-knowledge step by step as you relinquish habitual patterns of stress and the reactionary fight-or-flight responses to life situations. Pilates can inform *what we didn't know*—the skills that translate into daily living with joy and without pain, managing ourselves as whole, fully functional individuals, living life with "passion, purpose, and vitality"—envisioning something different in our life and perhaps the world.

What you are *not* thinking about while doing Pilates is as important as doing Pilates. Perhaps you start your Pilates session with your mind full of thoughts—events in your day, good, bad, or mundane, yesterday's regrets, tomorrow's worries. Then you begin to focus on the movement. You consciously choose to release your mind from needless distractions and open up to what is available within yourself—a cleansing and renewal of body, mind, and spirit, an "internal shower," as Joe would say.

You are arriving at your center.

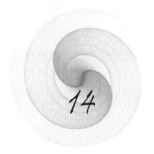

Chapter Fourteen

Centering

"A strong center is the focus of all the Pilates movements. It appears in different forms, but is always there. It is the foundation on which your new fitness, grace, and suppleness will be built."

Most of us didn't notice that centering as a path to health was introduced to us early on as a wall chart in our doctor's office. We all saw it. A human figure stripped of clothing and skin, revealing muscle and tissues, standing upright, its body aligned on an invisible center line, vertical in gravity. This body, as we all recall, seemed perfect in its form and was uniformly developed, i.e. a muscular representation of what appeared to be human potential. At the bottom of this wall chart were written the words *Physiologically Efficient Posture*. When one's spine uniformly aligned along gravity's vertical axis, the life-force-energy that governs our health systems and keeps us well is in good working order.

"A strong center is the focus of all the Pilates movements. It appears in different forms, but is always there. It is the foundation on which your new fitness, grace, and suppleness will be built." *The Pilates Method of Physical and Mental Conditioning,* Philip Friedman and Gail Eisen, (Doubleday and Company, 1980)

Finding our center and claiming ownership of it gives rise to physiological benefits too numerous to list, but one stands out, i.e. *getting free of pain.* More than half my clients have come to Pilates seeking relief from pain, both physical and mental. Why is that? Imbalance. An imbalanced musculoskeletal system puts pressure on joints that depletes circulation, causing inflammation affecting the nerves that give life energy to our organs and glands. Left unchecked, this is a downward spiral that can culminate in a myriad of problems.

During the time I was married to Susie, her Multiple Sclerosis symptoms became so severe that she needed a cane to support herself. When we went grocery shopping, she would have to grasp the shopping cart like a walker just to be able to navigate the grocery aisles. It was always a humbling experience for me. Often I choked back tears. Yet she would persevere, laughing and making light of the moment, not allowing the disability and pain to ruin her Saturday stroll through Whole Foods.

Years later we are divorced, yet we remain business partners and the best of friends; and we still shop for groceries together. Now I push the cart, and Susie walks the isles wearing high heels, arms crossed, turning her head side to side, scanning for items to snag and toss into our cart.

What happened to her, you ask? Pilates!

Following our divorce, and after a severe car accident that left her quite disabled and the loss of her job, Susie's depression and exhaustion almost got the best of her. Then, remembering the stories I had often told her, and wanting to stop her feelings of despair, when she noticed a new Pilates studio in her town of Littleton, Colorado, she decided to drop by to get acquainted. She wanted to find a studio run by a physical therapist who would be exceptionally patient, as her symptoms had become so bad that she couldn't decipher left from right.

Susie was no longer able to concentrate. Her memory was failing; it sometimes took her three hours to find her way home from the grocery store, five minutes away. She had a crack in her right patella, three bulging discs, thoracic outlet syndrome, and sciatic nerve damage. She was quickly losing her eyesight. On top of that, she was dealing with hemiplegic migraines—stabbing headaches with muscle weakness, and temporary paralysis in her legs, along with constant numbness in her hands and feet. I remember her telling me that she never went a day without severe pain.

It was a big step for Susie to contact the Pilates studio in Littleton. After meeting the owner of The Pilates Institute, Wendy Evans, a 'physio'—physical therapist and a Polestar Pilates certified practitioner, Susie felt such a connection that she committed to private sessions three to four times a week. This also put a financial strain on her, as she had no insurance and was not working.

"It was a real challenge to go to my appointments," she says. "There were days when my depression was too much, or I could barely walk; but I knew I did not want to be in the state I was in, and after my first appointment with Wendy, I knew that I liked the feeling I got from Pilates. I sensed a lightness and a feeling of euphoria. This was something I wanted in my life.

"I could tell that the sessions were working from the moment she taught me correct breathing from the core of my being. When I was in pain, I could breathe my way out of it. I also began to notice the difference in my driving. I was able to sit upright with my posture in a much more natural state and actually turn my head without severe pain in the neck. The most important change, though, was at night. When I couldn't sleep because my back pain was so severe, I lay in bed and did several pelvic bridges, then felt pain free enough to get to sleep.

"After several months, I was able to begin taking walks around the block and a few evening strolls. This was remarkable for me, as I used to tire just walking around my house or bringing in groceries.

"A year later and twenty pounds lighter, I feel and look fantastic. There are rare days when I still have pain and exhaustion, but I know now how to help the pain subside. And . . . I can walk a straight line without falling over. My creativity is even coming back to me!"

Once Susie found a very special Pilates teacher who could cater to her specific needs, balance returned to her life. Starting with correct breathing, she learned to concentrate and take

control of her body. Then, little by little, she found her center
and rediscovered her innate sense of balance. This was a
stunning achievement. Any body worker who understands the
biomechanics involved with Susie's condition will recognize
that her transformation is pretty miraculous!

**The metaphysical correlate to centering is balance, and the
connecting quality is discovery.**

How do we find our center?

Suppose for a moment that your life depends upon balance. For example, imagine that you are walking a tightrope
or high wire in the circus, without a net. There is no room
for distraction or imbalance. Out on the wire, more than technique is required. The aerialist must be completely focused
and completely centered. So it is with Pilates.

Progressing through Pilates movements with the understanding of this centerline, many Pilates students express
amazement at the tranquility they feel when done. These
tranquil feelings can return again and again, each time we
return to our center, feeling that good and happy with the
way life is going.

"The first requisite to happiness is fitness," Joe said.

So it is when you discover the center that governs your every
movement. Applying and understanding centering brings us
together as a whole—body, mind, and spirit—and alters our
illusion of separateness. When we are in balance, centered in
our body and our life, we are not in pain.

The converse is also true. When we are not internally
unified in body, mind, and spirit our outer perception of

separateness and pain is heightened. When we get out of balance, off center, we experience the intervention of gravity on our imbalanced structure.

It is known that gravity exerts the greatest stress on the body. No wonder, since gravity is the dominant force in the universe that holds stars together and prevents planets from colliding in their respective orbits. The question becomes how can we use gravity as a partner, rather than "fight gravity"?

Partnering with opposition, the relationship between up and down, in and out, front to back, and side to side is the key to accessing Pilates movement and to opening ourselves to possibilities, unlocking our joints, our spines, our minds. In its application and practice through Pilates, you befriend gravity and *rediscover balance as non-dominance.*

Through centering in gravity, Pilates liberates us by creating space in the body. It also decompresses the joints and frees our hips. More room for our organs; more space around our spinal discs; more 'head space' or what Joe alluded to as a sound mind capable of resolving issues: "Personal problems are clearly thought out and calmly met."

The practice of balancing the forces of gravity on and in our body—is a huge metaphor for the balance we bring to power and force in our life.

Thus Pilates is an exercise in mental and physical balance. This balancing act requires attention, cooperation, practice, and a sense of fulfilling purpose. These in turn lead us toward precision.

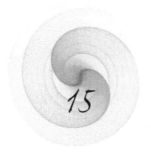

Chapter Fifteen

Precision

Pilates is a lifelong study. In doing the movements, under-standing *precisely what* you are doing is essential. At a deeper level, understanding *why* takes contemplation of your progress. Witness the slow change of seasons, as spring is born from winter's labor pains, or the human birth process—nine months from single cell to newborn infant. Each of us is a work in progress. A precept of Pilates precision is, the exact execution of each movement and the transition between each exercise in any endeavor worth doing well, precision comes to us through practice.

"Precision of motion and precision of placement creates a kind of bodily fine tuning that carries over into everyday life as grace and economy of movement." *The Pilates Method of Physical and Mental Conditioning*, Philip Friedman and Gail Eisen, (Doubleday and Company, 1980)

Precision implies perfection; but perfection is an abstract ideal (though the ego may argue this point). No day in life is perfect, nor are the circumstances in which you find yourself, nor is your performance in your next Pilates class. Yet in every circumstance, we can strive for and benefit from pursuing excellence, effortlessness, and grace, all aligning toward precision.

Moving toward precision—'a bodily fine tuning'—is adhering to a delicate balance; being in cooperation with what is.

Deane Juhan, author of *Jobs Body (Station Hill Press, 2002)*, reminds us that "unlike a cure, health has no clearly defined goal; it is open-ended, eternally unfinished, constantly challenged by changing conditions, always creating new levels of optimum performance and pleasure."

I recall working with brain-injured clients, resulting in closed head injuries from car accidents, who were referred to me for post-rehab by their doctors. Teaching them how to re-embody themselves through Pilates was part of their recovery process.

Part of my job was to document their progress from one Pilates session to the next—for example, from *unable to climb stairs without some dizziness*, to *able to climb stairs without use of handrail*. This is life-changing progress for a person with a brain injury. Eventually, such progress might translate into remembering details of a conversation, riding a bicycle, or other activities of daily living that had previously been beyond that person's ability. If this kind of improvement is possible for a brain-injured person, imagine what Pilates can do for those of us who are not so seriously challenged!

We have all experienced times as ordinary people faced with extraordinary circumstances. Some days especially remind us of just how imperfect life can be. Living our lives in unpredictability, what keeps us moving forward at times that seem distraught and hopeless? How good are we at this thing called life, with its intersections filled with crashes or near misses. Do we judge and then harshly react to circumstances beyond our control? Or hold an inner candle flame that never flickers?

Enter Grace, the metaphysical correlate to Precision. Grace is here defined as *seemingly effortless beauty of movement, form, and proportion*—truly a sight to behold, both in the Pilates studio and in life. When one is proficient in this more-than-exercise method of mental and physical conditioning, exuberance imbues our everyday dealings. Every Pilates teacher, student, and enthusiast knows the feeling one attains when in the flow of these choreographed movements. Feeling *fabulous* and *free* throughout your day is not an exaggeration—liberated from aches, pains, and preconceived notions of what you thought your life was limited to! If you are in the flow of life with grace, then your intentions become clearer and your life's passion becomes increasingly available.

The metaphysical correlate to precision is grace, and its connecting quality is effort with ease.

Think of your own life and times, or *even* a moment that was debilitating and seemingly insurmountable. Remember the feeling when you broke through—that's a fair analogy of the power Pilates can have in your life. This transcendence is evidenced by the stories told in this book.

As we move from being grounded in the Pilates principles: Breathing, Concentration, Control, Centering, Precision, and Flowing Movement, we discover a physical understanding of how to organize ourselves around a movement. Upon doing this and arriving at an outcome that goes beyond our expectation, *we must stop and recognize there is more to this than meets the eye!*

According to Deepak Chopra, grace is synonymous with the effortless flow of existence. "Move your body, exercise your body, and keep it moving. The more you dance with the universe, the more joy, vitality, energy, creativity, synchronicity, and harmony you will experience."

Thus precision is the acquired wisdom to set up the next movement and continue with grace. To move easily and *grace*fully with unbroken continuity, this brings us to flowing movement.

Chapter Sixteen

Flowing Movement

In the practice of Pilates exercises, 'flowing movement' is the vernacular for transitioning from one movement to the next without disrupting the *flow*—considered to be the most challenging and rewarding part of a Pilates 'workout.' Accessing sensory awareness within a Pilates movement, and then taking that to flow, has had a profound effect on me and those I have taught. The outcome we feel after a Pilates mat or equipment class may stake its claim as a partner in the greater experience of life. I recall a client saying after a Pilates class, "I cannot live my life without this!"

"In describing the essence of a Pilates movement, Romana Kryzanowska frequently speaks of 'flowing motion outward from a strong center.' Nothing should be stiff or jerky. Nothing should be too rapid or to slow. Smoothness and evenly flowing movement go hand in hand with control." *The Pilates Method of Physical and Mental Conditioning,* Philip Friedman and Gail Eisen, (Doubleday and Company, 1980)

Early in my Pilates training, during a weekend intensive, my then-business-partner and I were at dinner and I decided to have a glass of red wine to celebrate the end of a grueling weekend. The waitress set down the wine glass, thin stemmed with a large bulbous top, and I, slightly distracted, knocked it over as I reached for it, only to catch it again before it spilled or crashed on the floor. The look of amazement on my face was reflected back to me by my dinner partner as we both exclaimed in unison, "Pilates?!"

After a rigorous weekend of study in this method of physical and mental conditioning, my central nervous system was in sync, my bodily movements flowing naturally from my center. I didn't *think* about catching the glass—it was all one fluid movement. Time seemed to stop—as if the glass waited for me, and I simply made a precise, flowing catch.

What motivated me most of all to write this book was the curious, wondrous, and even miraculous sensations, like this, that I and others derive from the Pilates experience. Clients and colleagues share with me the same words that have come to my own mind when describing Pilates: lightness, inner peace, connectedness.

"Everyone experiences flow from time to time and will recognize its characteristics: People typically feel strong, alert, in effortless control, unselfconscious, and at the peak of their abilities. Both the sense of time and emotional problems seem to disappear, and there is an exhilarating feeling of transcendence," says author Mihaly Csikszentmihalyi, Ph.D. in the book *Flow: The Psychology of Optimal Experience,* (Harper Perennial, 1991)

More than seventy years ago, Joseph Pilates was teaching the idea that mastery of flowing movement led one to happiness. If you are in a state of happiness, not only can you ward off illness and invite health, but you will also feel more in control of your life.

I believe this is why clients keep coming back and why Pilates has flourished across the planet. In times like these, people want to *feel good and live with intention.*

The metaphysical correlate to flowing movement is synchronicity, and the connecting quality is intention.

After practicing Pilates breath, technique, and choreography on the equipment or mat, putting these elements together results in a felt sense of familiarity. Synchronicity of movement introduces an exhilarating quickening of mind-body dynamics, reinforcing our resolve and enlivening our purpose. The daily grind of the ups and downs of life aren't hanging in the balance at this moment and, gaining momentum from what once was limitation, we are renewed with the joy of being in alignment, once again, with our intention. When we grasp 'going with the flow,' getting things accomplished in our lives is not happenstance or coincidental but an indicator that we are in rhythm with life happening.

Today, we have a deeper understanding of the "unspoken" metaphysical benefits of Pilates. As we have seen in the remarkable stories in this book of lives transformed, Pilates offers a path to health through increasing self-awareness.

Quality of attention, being in the now, self-knowledge, discovery, effort with ease, and intention—these are the connections that bridge the gap between action, *how* we do Pilates, and thought, *why* we do Pilates. The following chart considers the six principles as a whole, along with their corresponding metaphysical benefits:

Pilates Principle	Connection	Metaphysical Correlation
BREATHING How does the quality of an individual's breath pattern influence the quality of their life?	*Quality of Attention*	AWARENESS OF SELF I am aware of myself and my relationship with my environment
CONCENTRATION Why is improved attention on self a valuable experience? How does this activity serve me? How does this new observation influence my perception of life?	*Being in the Now*	PRESENT MOMENT AWARENESS I learn something from this action and I can change and grow at any time
CONTROL Is there a correlation between controlling your movements and being in control of your life? What state of mind do you find yourself in to be in control of your life?	*Self Knowledge*	CONSCIOUS CHANGE I can freely choose my state of mind noting its conditioned patterns and constructs
CENTERING What is a predictable outcome if you aren't centered? Do you feel centered when you are seated, standing or walking?	*Discovery*	BALANCE I notice my inner outer relationship(s) with the environment so I can function at my greatest potential
PRECISION How does haphazard movement and happenstance thinking disempower your life?	*Effort with Ease*	GRACE I can embody a new sense of fitness, evoking body and mind balance
FLOWING MOVEMENT Can going with the flow of life be a new perceived reality that attracts what you want?	*Intention*	SYNCHRONICITY I am co-creating through Source, transforming my life to all things good that serve me

The "Metaphysical Correlation" column of the chart tells what you are learning during, or how you might feel after, a Pilates session. *Awareness of self, present moment awareness, conscious choice, balance, grace, and synchronicity* are indicators of our gain beyond the movement, aligning us with a higher state of consciousness.

Each step, from left to right, gives rise to the next. The left column, "Pilates Principle," represents the process of being in the inquiry. The right column "Metaphysical Correlation" proposes an answer to this inquiry in the form of affirmation. Many of us have used affirmations as one of our daily practices to improve our lives. And the "Connection," the center column, is how you arrived at the positive outcome or "unspoken" benefit derived from your Pilates experience.

As you read the table, consider how Pilates can deepen your understanding of yourself. I encourage you to **notice** how you feel after doing Pilates, why you pursue it, and what shows up in your life. **Notice within you that which wasn't present when you started**. Perhaps this is what Joe meant when he talked about "the resulting sensation of uplift."

As a teacher, and I feel sure many other teachers reading this would agree, the greatest thrill is the quality of beauty we see in our clients when they are achieving the deeper expression of the movement. Many times, in many studios, nationally and internationally, you can hear the kudos expressed to our clients, an exuberant, joyous shout of: "THAT'S BEAUTIFUL— BEAUTIFULLY DONE!!"

And for those Pilates enthusiasts—client or student—reading this: You may experience a resulting sense of peace, glimpsing an inner truth—that unity cannot be fought for and won, only felt, one individual at a time.

As part of his vision, Joe said to expect "spiritual enhancements" in your life. This is now understood in tangible 21st century vernacular. Pilates is a life affirming practice which evokes a return to purpose and passion. *A return to life!*

Chapter Seventeen

The Role of Equipment

Having explored the six core principles of Contrology, it is important to understand the role of equipment in today's Pilates world.

Joe called his innovative equipment "*apparatus.*" Apparatus, by definition, implies something different in association with 'exercise equipment', and the use of may take an individual beyond a mere 'workout.'

Apparatus is defined, in part as "to make ready, preparation." Pilates 'equipment' was intended to make ready in preparation for the mat work.

The mat work is more familiar to consumers today by reading 'how-to-do' books on the subject and taking 'mat classes' made available through gyms and health clubs. Mat classes are usually at no extra cost to health club members, while equipment workouts have an up charge in addition to membership dues. While it is not unusual in these economic times to minimize our overhead and go with what is economical, *this unfortunately leaves a misunderstood gap within the Pilates experience.* **The equipment and the mat work go hand in hand.**

This is the distinction of your neighborhood Pilates studio facility. The apparatus (equipment) used in practice there will assist and support you, preparing you for the mat work. And the sequence of exercises on any given piece of equipment will *deepen your knowledge and will assist in opening your body to execute the levels of mat work.*

More so, from a therapeutic perspective, the apparatuses are designed to support the body and close the kinetic chain. Most often they employ a spring connected to a solid surface and the individual's hand or foot or both—a guidance system assisting your movement of an arm or leg to and fro (hence the inception of bedsprings used on hospital beds circa WWI), to create a felt sense of connection to the movement. The springs act as a conduit to connect, coordinate, and inform the relationship of body and mind. This, in its day, was referred to as "marrying the apparatus" and can inform a person's alignment, misalignment, strength, or weakness. This partnership guides the individual toward correct and healthful alignment, leading to a quickening on the mat!

What does a typical Pilates session involve? Most Pilates exercise offers an average of three to eight repetitions and within an hour, based on the skill set of the group session, can indulge in thirty-four or more movements just by lying on a mat. Today, this may be a more acceptable and manageable approach when time constraints seem to run our lives. More so, this hour retreat offers a boost to our immune system, and balance within the day to day responsibilities, which may support and refresh one's perspective of the week.

There is a notion in certain circles of the Pilates community that *the mat work is the work,* and mastery would be the intended pursuit of it. *To that end, how you arrive there is a personal journey.* Some of you may be asking, "Do I need the equipment to have a positive movement experience on the mat?" First and foremost, check with your physician or physical therapist to determine if you have any spinal or muscular condition that would prevent you. Secondly, find a Pilates teacher, like a coach, who will give attention to your personal condition, leading you into sensory awareness, and modifying your movement with props to support the body and to assist, stabilize, and inform. An adept Pilates teacher suggests mastery of knowing his/her students' needs. *This partnership between student and teacher is critical for a positive movement experience, particularly for the novice, and* learning from a video/DVD may be counterproductive to your desired outcome.

In my initial training, when being overwhelmed by the magnitude of some 500 exercises possible within the brilliance of Joe's method, I posed this question to First Generation Pilates teacher Romana Kryzanowska, a dedicated disciple of Joe's, "What would you recommend out of all this that would be essential to the clients' health and wellbeing?" She responded, "Mat work and footwork on the reformer."

Here is what I attest to . . . *Pilates is a meaningful practice—on a mat or on equipment—and with the guidance of a knowledgeable, compassionate teacher, is life changing.*

Part Four

Pilates for Our Times

Pilates for Our Times

"We are exiting the era of survival of the fittest and entering an era of survival of the wisest." —Survival of the Wisest, *Dr. Jonas Salk, (Harper & Row, 2003)*

In my initial training I was taught to teach who is in front of me and to ask, *What is it that I can offer an individual?—or What might be missing in their awareness to improve their personal condition?* In my experience, the greater majority who showed up were individuals far from the buffed persona of an athlete; not someone with a bent on getting fit or in shape by the standard set forth from a multibillion-dollar mega advertising campaign. No. These were regular folks looking for something that could help their present condition and help them better face the challenges of today's world. As the stories in this book have shown, and the stories of the many thousands of people who have transformed their lives, *Pilates can be a self-help therapy—a health maintenance system intended to bring forth the self-healing potential we all hold innate in our being.*

This book was intended to discover the essence of what we experience in the practice of Pilates in the 21st century, and open ourselves up to the possibility that the outcome is something greater than just a 'workout.' Let us take a look at today's Pilates community and its ability to transform lives, starting with my own.

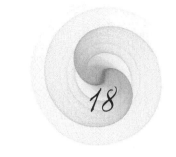

Chapter Eighteen

My Personal Journey

I am so grateful to Joseph Pilates for his inspired work, and to the Pilates Elders who studied directly with him and kept his teachings alive. These teachings, along with my studies in holistic health and the years of studying and teaching Pilates, are all truly responsible for inspiring me to write this book. What I have learned and am now putting into words is that what we are really doing in Pilates is discovering who we are, at a core level, and that everything is connected within us— body, mind, and spirit. This renewed knowledge can guide us in the face of circumstances that appear beyond our control.

My experience of Pilates started in 1991 with meeting my first teachers, Amy and Rachel, fondly known as "the Taylor sisters," founders of The Pilates Center of Boulder. At this meeting in their center, seeing the revolutionary Pilates spring-based equipment for the first time, I was arrested by a strong feeling of, "I have been here before." This déjà vu was so strong and disorienting that it brought tears to my eyes, and my newfound teachers concernedly asked if I was all right. I couldn't speak for the alchemy I was feeling, a strange mix of fear and bliss. Nor did I realize then (now twenty years into the future) they would offer me Joe's letter of 1939, a historical archival document, essentially their mission statement, to bring greater relevancy to this book.

I enrolled and received my certification as a Pilates teacher in 1993. After a rigorous fifteen months of combined learning, observing, and teaching, I remember during my final exam, the practicum, I've never been so nervous and it showed. Amy called out in a compassionate voice, "Where's the joy?" She revived my sense of purpose. I was among its first graduates, and I have been a practicing Pilates teacher ever since.

In my graduating class was a gracious woman named Wendy LeBlanc-Arbuckle. When I met her, I was immediately drawn to her extraordinary spirit and wisdom. To me she felt like a sister, but I soon learned that she was also to be a mentor who would awaken in me recognition of the truth that Pilates is not merely a form of exercise, but a means of connecting to the Life Force that resides within us all. *"Let's keep discovering how to live with passion, purpose, and vitality!"* was her motto.

Drawing inspiration from her background as a longtime yoga and somatic movement teacher, Wendy shared with me her inquiry into the universal principles that inform all movement. Her words resonate to this day . . . *"Remember that the body doesn't care if we are practicing yoga, Pilates, Alexander,*

or whatever. What it responds to is accessing its deep relation-
ship with gravity and breath."

In 1999, I was invited by Wendy and her husband Michael
(co-founder of Peak Pilates, an internationally recognized
Pilates equipment company) to join them in Austin, Texas
to be Associate Director of the distinctive Core Connections®
Pilates Teacher Training Program. This program was grounded
in the classical repertoire and standing on the shoulders of
Joseph Pilates' philosophy of whole body health and wellbeing. They asked me to assist in certain aspects of its delivery.
During the next year and a half, through Wendy's tutelage,
I discovered in Pilates a vast knowledge of how the body,
mind, and spirit relate, and how to *embrace human potential*
through the empowerment of self.

Building upon my early Pilates training, now I was exploring a holistic approach, in how someone who was sensing
their movement was just as important to their development
as their goal to "learn how to do the exercises." This helped
me build a new foundation on which my teaching of Pilates
principles is fostered: *awareness*, cultivating self-knowledge,
and an ability to be self-healing.

Coming from my longtime holistic roots and appreciating
the value of preventative healthcare, it was a natural progression to acknowledge Pilates as "energy medicine."

Energy medicine is a modern field with age-old roots.
It borrows from traditional healing methods and integrates
them into modern settings and perspectives as a compliment
to western medical care. It can address physical, mental, and
emotional ailments as well as peak performance.

It is my view that Pilates creates a higher, energetic frequency to occur within an individual client and that client's teacher. Energies, both electromagnetic and subtle, align with the dynamic infrastructure of the physical body. The quality of those energies in terms of flow, balance, and harmony make up our physiology—*the quality of our health.* When the body is depleted of these energies it is more difficult to manage emotions, think positive thoughts, and stay healthy. *Where thought goes, energy follows.* An energetic shift to flow, balance, and harmony are an outcome from Pilates. The Pilates experience renders a depletion of heaviness and ushers in a higher vibrational frequency—a feeling of lightness. Thus the quality of life evolves, one individual at a time.

"Structural integrity and vibratory or energetic, or informational integrity go hand in hand—one cannot influence the structural system without influencing the energetic/informational system and vice versa." *Energy Medicine: The Scientific Basis*, James L. Oschman, (Elsevier Limited, 2000)

Twenty-first century science says that mind and body are integrated and entwined with the world at large. It isn't that the mind is housed in the brain within the body. The mind is in the body—literally in every cell of the body, and acts as one interdependent whole—a thinking body. Illuminating our understanding of this 'field' from a health and healing perspective, rehabilitation expert Dr. Carol Davis tells us that "Just because we cannot perceive a part of all that is real (the non-material, the non-local, the invisible) does not mean that it does not exist and is not present interacting in meaningful ways with what we do perceive."

This renewed sensory awareness—*what we didn't know that we didn't know*—can quicken our resolve in the face of circumstance that appear to be beyond our control. In this vein, I have a particular talent working with clients who are re-covering from an injury or long-standing problem. *Healing is an inside job* for those *ready and willing* to take control of possibility, and that the Pilates experience can be a light at the end of a tunnel.

After completing my agreement at Pilates Center of Austin, I returned to Fort Collins to resume my business. On September 11, 2001, though I was far removed from the epicenter like countless millions of Americans, I was stunned by the enormity of the senseless acts and loss of lives. In the following months, I gradually realized that the tragedy of 9/11 had coincided with the beginning of a *downward spiraling* in my own life. In a few short months I would experience the lowest point in my entire life.

My business plan collapsed, and for the next two years, I fought against the looming threat of bankruptcy. In the end, I could not hold out. Matters worsened when my wife suffered the unexpected onset of multiple sclerosis (MS). (Her own Pilates 'miracle' is recounted in Chapter Fourteen.) The stress in our lives escalated to unbearable at times. Even though we worked with a counselor, trying to salvage what was left of our marriage, in the end, my wife decided that a divorce was the healthiest choice we could make. Sadly, I had to agree.

I was fifty years old, bankrupt, divorced, negotiating to stop or stall a foreclosure on my house, and dependent on unemployment checks. My physical body expressed only pain. All the life, the love, the energy, the hope, and the expectations of my world had collapsed. On every level, in every category, I needed help.

I was fortunate enough to find a medical clinic devoted to helping low income people. "There, but for the grace of God, go I." I thought, as I sat in a chair waiting for my name to be called out. The room was overflowing with destitute people. Although my heart felt compassion, a deep fear surfaced. Am I one of these people? What has happened to me? Why am I here?

I was scanning the room, when something on the wall caught my eye. I squinted at it, then stood up and navigated my pained, unwilling body over to it for a closer look. These words stared back at me:

> *Life is either a daring adventure or nothing. To keep our faces toward change and behave like free spirits in the presence of fate is strength undefeatable.*
>
> *—Helen Keller*

A teary-eyed peace came over me. *Maybe,* I thought, *maybe* **this** *moment, and the rest of my life, is already in perfect order.*

"Gary Calderone?" a woman queried. As I turned around, my body winced in pain, the same pain that had brought me to this place, the same pain that had crippled my abilities to do my work. The world slowed way down, and I felt a knowing that I was at a crossroads of some kind in my life.

For me, what was about to happen was an experience in reinventing myself from a condition that does not define me.

Using the last of my resources, and re-connecting with what I had learned in Austin, over the next several months, twice each week, I drove more than an hour each way to get to a Pilates session at The Pilates Center in Boulder. Well, it was either Pilates or prescription painkillers. Pilates became my painkiller.

Returning to this place, *now humbled in the presence of my Pilates teacher, enabled me to do what I had forgotten.* In the process of my downward spiral, I had forgotten what I had for years taught others. The problem that was interfering with my health could be resolved or healed with awareness and Pilates.

When it finally dawned on me that the place I needed to be was a Pilates studio, and not some hospital bed, I began to 'return to life.' In three months, my life turned around.

An inner knowing, a belief that I was capable of healing myself, allowed me to reject the thought that I needed a wheel-chair. And even though my left leg felt as if it were someone else's leg, unfamiliar and non-responsive for almost a year after the onset of the problem, the *access to sensory awareness* I had gathered from my apprenticeship in Austin brought me back in touch with my movement and life purpose. As I was re-connected with my deeper Pilates practice, my left leg was no longer an issue.

Breakthrough occurs in the opening you create for yourself.

I am fondly reminded, as I can best recall, of Marianne Williamson's words, a pioneer and author of spiritual consciousness:

'What did or didn't happen in your past is not the determining factor in the arch of what is possible in your life.

Possibility is not just an abstract obscure notion, but the yearning response of a force in the universe—greater than ourselves—ceaselessly expanding to evolve your present state of mind, not the failures, mistakes, and disappointments of memories and reminders of the haunting, distant past, noticing that life doesn't usually progress, if ever, in an uninterrupted straight line of moving forward in one's life.'

—Marianne Williamson quote; *The Age of Miracles, Embracing the New Midlife,* Marianne Williamson, (Hay House, 2008)

And so it is, that a rekindled spirit has emerged (along with a revitalized body) with a passion and privilege to share with you my journey . . . it is my hope that the words herein expressed in some way contribute deeply to yours.

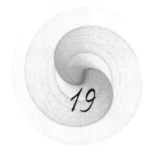

Chapter Nineteen

Vision Forward

"This world of ours is in turmoil and no one is positive of its outcome, and it is now more than ever before, more practicable and sensible, to be in a perfect state of health, both in body and in mind, in order to more successfully confront the problems continually arising."
(JHP; 1939 letter to clients)

Why now, decades after Joseph's time, are so many people turning to Pilates? Like me, many have come to the practice as a last chance: a last chance before surgery, a last chance before pharmaceuticals, or a last chance before resigning to a life of limitation, disappointment, and broken dreams.

As we have seen through the many moving stories in this book, Pilates heals by fostering the individual spirit. The results are astonishing. As in my own recovery, a great majority of clients find out within three to six months of starting Pilates that their limiting thoughts are a thing of the past.

Going beyond exercise trends, this book has sought to illuminate the unique trinity of body, mind, and spirit—*this felt sense of something greater* that makes this decades-old health technology purposeful and relevant for these times. Pilates does more than help us self-heal. Pilates offers a new paradigm to help us confront a changing world and circumstances that seem beyond our control as we move forward through the 21st century.

Much like how Joseph Pilates felt about the world he lived in, many of us today may feel lost amid the turmoil of our world—the dissonance and erratic pulse of life, international conflict, an uncertain economy, and the ever-looming issues of health. Many may be searching for something permanent and meaningful in an ever-changing landscape of science, religion, and cultural values.

Joe's writings are a roadmap toward a reawakened life. Joe was essentially saying to anyone who would listen, *do my exercises, you'll be healthier, happier . . . you'll change your life . . . and better to be able to face the challenges of the world.*

Joe said, "The *mind, when housed within a healthy body, possesses a glorious sense of power.*" Is this his call to action from our deepest aspect to reconnect?

As we move through the 21st century, our ability to solve problems will be pushed to the limits, and the systems that are familiar, that are no longer working, will fall apart against the pressure of change. How we grow our 'wisdom from the ages' is evident by the teachers that came before us, known as the 1st Generation Pilates Elders (whose personal stories and contributions to the practice are highlighted in the Appendix to this book). These instructors, and their unique approaches to serve all types of bodies, individually represent that *there is more than one interpretation on how Pilates is done and that one size does not fit all.*

I once observed a Pilates class being taught to a mixed group of abilities where the Pilates Elder was inviting everyone to be in sync with everyone else. I had a profound revelation from a quote by Werner Erhard: *It has to work for everyone or it works for no one.* Experiencing the cooperation required to honor the individual—*what makes an exercise work for one, different for another*—observing this, *that one person's success is the community's success,* provides a glimpse of what makes living as a community work on our planet. It is my opinion that this *unspoken* reciprocal relationship is perhaps the innate calling answered by thousands of Pilates teachers worldwide.

The preservation of Joe and Clara's work and wisdom has taken on different forms through various organizations and institutions worldwide. What is important to note is that the intention of these entities is the betterment of humankind, keeping alive Joe's idea that will assist millions of individuals in realizing their potential, arriving at self-awareness as healthy individuals unified by a balanced, coordinated trinity of body, mind, and spirit.

Our common link with each other—by creating guidelines of safety and excellence in the teaching methods—is that we all care. Like all diverse communities, we may struggle with how to transcend beyond these standards and ideals to reach a greater understanding of our principles and values. We can't move forward into the future while holding on to the past notion of *how it should be*. Those in leadership roles will be challenged to honor our differences and listen for what the Pilates collective is asking. *How can we be moved, touched, and inspired by the greatness of the work, seek to learn from and grow with one another, and, to that end, progress the Pilates community toward higher principles and wisdom?*

Thus, how do we stand on the shoulders of Joseph Pilates, staying in the inquiry of what is possible, as we move into the 21st century and beyond?

Here are a few suggestions:

- As a practitioner:
    - *Participating in a collective practice that offers both mat and equipment classes from a Certified Pilates Teacher to develop a coordinated and uniquely balanced trinity of body, mind, and spirit.*
    - *Being open to investigating new paths toward optimal health.*

- As a teacher:
    - Reviving traditional teaching methods and adapting evolved techniques and equipment.
    - Reviewing new science technology and acknowledging intuitive exploration.
    - Building incremental awareness within one person and one thought at a time.

- As a student:
  - Educating yourself, connecting with your body, and directing your attention inward.
  - Realizing that Pilates is a sustainable resource that helps you to thrive in difficult times.

Joe and Clara would be proud to see the expanse of their influence and wisdom into our future.

Mary Bowen, a student of Joe and Clara, perhaps summarizes it best:

"Pilates changes lives. Pilates resurrects. Pilates challenges people to connect and grow through the body—but not only the body . . .

Pilates is practical. Pilates strengthens. Pilates aligns. Pilates enlivens. Pilates heals. Pilates inspires and leads to more of oneself. Pilates is helpful and useful in every aspect of life for as long as one lives. Joe and Clara knew that. They lived that and gave their lives to share it with the rest of us. Thank you, Joe and Clara."

Remember—*it is always the development, brilliance, and genius of you, the individual.* Change doesn't come through the country, the tribe, or the group. Change begins and ends with the individual. We must always value and foster the individual journey, the life lived in a certain way that inspires and awakens. As you improve your connection to health through awareness and consciousness, not only does your life improve—what is possible expands.

So begins your Pilates journey.

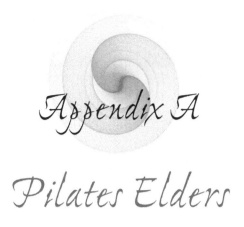

Appendix A

Pilates Elders

As there are many paths to healing, so are there many paths to Pilates. The disciples who studied personally with Joe and Clara—those still alive and those who have passed—have come to be known today as 1st Generation or Elders, and they have left their indelible marks on the thousands, if not millions, who follow their interpretations of what Joe and Clara left for us: the future generations of Pilates teachers, students, and enthusiasts. The following is a compilation of biographical information to help us understand these Elders, their reasons for embracing Pilates in their times, and how their knowledge may translate into our own. For those Elders no longer with us, embellishments from others who knew them are expressed in their honor. And to be equitable with biographical information, websites, where applicable, are given for the readers who desire to know more.

The Elders

Romana Kryzanowska came to New York as a young woman to study dance under George Balanchine at the School of American Ballet. Balanchine introduced her to Joe and Clara Pilates in 1941, after she had injured her ankle. Joe promised her that he would heal her ankle in five sessions. When she found herself recovering after only three sessions, she became a lifelong devotee of Contrology. Years later, after Joe's passing, Clara selected Romana to take over the direction of the original New York Pilates Studio. Although that studio closed in 1989, Romana continues to teach and train other Pilates teachers to this day. She has always emphasized the original philosophy and techniques of Joseph Pilates and is regarded by many as the keeper of the 'true' or classical Pilates way.

Rachel and Amy Taylor, owners of The Pilates Center and protégé of Romana, offer these insights: "My sister Amy and I studied several years with Romana in the late 1980's and we were "certified" by her to teach Pilates at the very beginning of her teacher training program. She is an amazingly energetic, compassionate, and demanding teacher whose every word and gesture embodied her love of Mr. Pilates and devotion to his method. She stated many times that she was teaching "Uncle Joe's" work exactly the way he taught it and had no desire to ever create anything beyond or outside of that—it was more than enough. We learned from her "to trust the method" and therefore Mr. Pilates and his visions of health and beauty as a body-mind-spirit experience as well as making a difference in the world, one body at a time."

www.purepilates.net

Ron Fletcher began dancing with the Martha Graham Dance Company in New York during the mid-1940s. When a knee injury threatened to end his career, he sought help from Joe and Clara Pilates. Contrology exercises eventually allowed him to return to dancing. In 1967, shortly before Joe's death, Ron came back to the Pilates Studio to continue training in Contrology. In 1971, with Clara's blessing, he opened the Ron Fletcher Studio for Body Contrology in Beverly Hills, California. Before long, his clientele included such well-known Hollywood figures as Candice Bergen, Ali McGraw, Judith Krantz, and Barbra Streisand. Ron sums up the Pilates movement experience as, "Movement should be approached like life—with enthusiasm, joy and gratitude—for movement is life, and life is movement and we get out of it what we put into it".

Pat Guyton, a protégée of Ron says, "Ron teaches integration of breath and movement to create a total experience of body, mind, and spirit. He calls his approach a "marvelous organic recipe" that draws inspiration from his years with Martha Graham and other master dancers as well as the techniques of Joseph Pilates. Ron continues teaching to this day."

www.fletcherpilates.com

Eve Gentry, whose early training was in ballet and Spanish dance, in 1929 left her parents' home in Southern California to pursue her dance passion. Her first exposure to modern dance was in San Francisco with Ann Munstock. Later, in New York City, she studied with Martha Graham, Doris Humphrey, Helen Tamiris, and at Ballet Arts and the Joffrey Ballet. She was also a member of the Hanya Holm Company from 1936 to 1942. In 1940, Gentry and three other dancers founded the Dance Notation Bureau. She was, in fact, the first American dancer to teach Labanotation in this country. While continuing her own solo career, Gentry directed her own Dance Company from 1944 to 1968. Eve was also a charter faculty member of the High School for Performing Arts, NYC and the New York University School of the Arts. Most significant in this context, she served as teacher and associate with Joseph Pilates himself in New York from 1942 to 1968. Relocating to Santa Fe, New Mexico in 1968, Gentry established a Dancer's Studio and a Pilates Studio. Both studios flourished in the following decades. She was also the Movement Technique Instructor for the Apprentice Program at the Santa Fe Opera for five seasons. In addition, Gentry choreographed and danced in Stravinsky's *La Rossignol* in 1969 and 1970, and at the age of 63 danced in the world premiere of Villa-Lobos' *Yerma* (choreographed by José Limon).

During her more than fifty year career, Ms. Gentry was a dancer, teacher (Pilates and dance), coach, and choreographer for countless stage, film, and television projects. In 1979, Bennington College honored her with the Pioneer of Modern Dance award, and in 1989 she was chosen as a "Santa Fe Living Treasure."

Over the years, Eve's students continued to come from all parts of the country to work with her. As only one among many testaments to her influence, Evelyn Lear (celebrated soprano at the Metropolitan Opera and La Scala) offered this: "Eve Gentry was a revelation in my life . . . . Under her loving and knowing guidance, I now lead a life free of pain and filled with total energy." Michele Larsson, a protégée of Eve recalls, " . . . there is one thing that stands out, Eve was incredibly generous with her knowledge and totally supportive of our experimenting (with her methods)."

Carola Trier was a professional dancer and acrobatic contortionist who came to Joseph Pilates in the early 1940s after severely injuring her back. To her amazement, Joe's exercises enabled her to completely heal and regain her mobility, and from then on she was an avid devotee. By the late 1950s, Carola became the first of Joe and Clara's students to open her own Pilates studio in New York, where she specialized in rehabilitating the injuries associated with dancing. She maintained close ties with Joe and Clara until their deaths, and went on to train a number of influential 'next-generation' Pilates teachers. She passed away in the year 2000 at the age of eighty-seven.

Jillian Hessel, a protégé of Carola, shares an insight. "I also remember Carola's one–on-one specialized work with a polio victim who was paralyzed in one leg and who exercised wearing a brace. Carola had an instinctive nurturing and gentle side that prompted her to dole out extra attention when someone was emotionally upset or injured. I will never forget what Carola said to me that day. 'You have to love helping people, and then when you really help them, you'll find the satisfaction most rewarding.'"

Kathleen Stanford Grant is another important keeper of the Pilates flame. Like many of Joe's students, Kathy Grant was a dancer before she began her training in Pilates. As a child in the late 1920's, Kathy Grant studied at the Boston conservatory of Music. She was a chorus girl at New York's famous Zanzibar Club, and worked in a number of Broadway and off Broadway productions, television programs, and toured in the United States, Europe, Africa, and the Middle East, and as a choreographer and co-director for a number of dance companies. Kathy Grant had injured her knee in a fall, and was hoping that Pilates could help her rehabilitate her knee so she could return to dancing. She became a longtime student of Joe Pilates, and she was one of only two people to receive official Pilates certification through a federally subsidized program of instruction approved of and supervised by Joe himself at the New York State Division of Vocational Rehabilitation. (Lolita San Miguel, discussed below, was the other.) Kathy taught at Carola Trier's studio and later managed the Pilates studio in the famous Henri Bendel department store from 1972 until it closed in 1988. After the studio closed, Kathy continued teaching Pilates workshops and seminars around the world. Kathy Grant taught Pilates on the faculty of the Department of Dance at the Tisch School of the Arts, New York University; Alpers, Segel, and Gentry, the authors of *The Everything Pilates Book* (Adams Media Corporation, 2002).

Cara Reeser, a protégée of Kathy, shares her fond memory: "Kathy's legacy lives in the hearts and work of many of her student's including myself. Twenty years later I am profoundly touched by the work and mentorship that I received from Kathy. Not a day goes by without her voice reminding me how to guide my clients, expand my practice, and joyously and confidently live and conduct my life; as a teacher, mentor, mover, and dreamer."

Lolita San Miguel, Director of Ballet Concierto de Puerto Rico, was the other student who received official Pilates certification through the vocational program supervised by Joe himself at the New York State Division of Vocational Rehabilitation. She studied with both Joe Pilates and Carola Trier in the 1960s, and went on to found, in 1977, the Ballet

Concierto de Puerto Rico in San Juan, the island's premier classical ballet company, and to develop a distinguished career there as a dancer, choreographer, director, and educator. She has become one of the leading cultural figures in Puerto Rico. In 2000, she retired from Ballet Concierto and founded Pilates Y Mas in order to teach, train, and certify teachers in the Pilates Method.

Lolita inspired and accomplished 21st century visions for Pilates by suggesting that a mentorship program, known as Passing the Torch, be established for Pilates professionals to deepen their knowledge. She also made it her mission to erect the Joseph Pilates Memorial in Germany.

Brent Anderson, a protégé, offers this insight,"Lolita, mi querida amiga, truly lives and exemplifies Joe's vision. She demonstrates to all of us how to live a life balanced between work, play and rest (well 2 out of 3 isn't bad). She exudes health and as Joe said "Health is the first requirement to being happy" and Lolita is happy. Most importantly I love the spiritual side of the work that she embraces and shares with all through her mere presence. Her posture alone speaks volumes. Thanks for the example!!!"

www.lolitapilates.com

Bruce King was another early student. In fact, he had an apartment near the Pilates' storeroom at the back of the building on Eighth Avenue where the original Pilates studio was located. A professional dancer, Bruce trained for many years with Joseph and Clara Pilates and was a member of the Merce Cunningham Company, the Alwyn Nikolais Company, and his own Bruce King Dance Company. He served as artist-in-residence at various universities and taught regularly at Adelphi University and the American Academy of Dramatic Arts. In the mid-1970s, King opened his own studio at 160 W. 73rd Street in New York City, and also traveled extensively teaching Pilates workshops around the country. He died in New York on January 01, 1993 in New York City at the age of sixty-seven.

Mary Bowen a student of Bruce King, tells us, "until he died, [his teaching] was the closest to what is called "classical Pilates" and a great teacher of the value and lack of boredom in repetition. With Bruce it was always the same way, the same forms in the same order. I was fifty when I started with him. I had the patience by then for his kind of quest for perfection through repetition. I could always find newness in it."

www.pilates-marybowen.com

Mary Bowen was an actress/comedienne/singer with a low back problem when she luckily found Joe and Clara in 1959 from a newspaper article. She spent six and a half years twice a week in their training. Joe was seventy-six when Mary began with him. She was twenty-nine. Also in 1959 she began studying psychoanalysis (Carl Jung's analytical psychology). These two, Pilates and the Psyche, evolved into the major roots of her life. By 1971 she had become a practicing Jungian psychoanalyst with offices in New York City, Killingworth, Connecticut, and New York City, extending her analytic work to Northampton, Massachusetts in 1975. Also by 1975 she had become a Pilates teacher. Mary sets a great example in having continued weekly private lessons in Pilates for herself, forty-nine years now. Mary's unique contribution to the Pilates community is Pilates Plus Psyche where she evolved and teaches a combination of Pilates and Jungian Analytical Psychology taking on the whole person, both the conscious and the unconscious. Through teaching Jungian typology, she helps teachers and clients to better understand their own difficulties and limitations through knowledge of their typology. This knowledge can be transforming, leading to better acceptance and tolerance of oneself and others. In Mary's own words (2009): "Practicing Pilates for fifty years with a lesson every week for myself is tantamount to a lifetime of Pilates, with no end yet in sight at seventy-nine. Teaching now for thirty-four years, my practice and understanding of the Pilates Method has evolved and changed as I evolve and change—always for the better."

Wendy Leblanc-Arbuckle invites Mary each year to the Pilates Center of Austin to share her wisdom with clients, students and Pilates teachers alike."Knowing and working with Mary over the years has deeply affected my life and teaching. Mary's gift is the space of loving presence, childlike joy, and samurai spirit with timeless wisdom she embodies. In being with Mary, we give birth to the depth of our authentic selves."

www.pilates-marybowen.com

Mary Pilates has been doing Pilates for over seventy years as of this writing (2009) and at age eighty-five is still in good physical condition. The niece of Joe and Clara Pilates, Mary grew up doing Pilates, though as a child she did not take it seriously, and she was often present and observant when Joe and his brother Fred, her father, experimented and tinkered with the equipment, most of which Fred built, as he was a carpenter by trade. Around 1935, Fred moved his family to St. Louis, Missouri, where he opened his own Pilates studio. In 1940, when she was eighteen, Mary traveled by bus from St. Louis to New York where she lived with Joe and Clara and became an apprentice in the New York Studio for several years, where she assisted Joe and Clara with their clients and students. She returned to St. Louis, married, becoming Mary LeRiche, and in 1959 moved to Margate, Florida, where she still lives. Retired for more than twenty years from the factory job she once held, Mary has become quite active in her local Pilates community. She adheres strictly to the methods as Joe and Clara taught them to her, and has founded and is Executive Director of Original Pilates® Instruction. She is also associated with Parkland Pilates, of Coral Springs, Florida, having certified Fran Perel, the proprietor. She has also been a close friend and mentor to MJ Mermer and is a regular at her MJ Pilates Studio in Coral Springs, Florida, also certified.

Kevin Bowen, co-founder of the Pilates Method Alliance interviewed Mary and recalls an impressive demonstration. "I of course remember Mary very well. She was very unassuming, quiet, but with a strong sense of self. She spoke about her 'Uncle' Joe very fondly. She had been sent to live with Joe and Clara when she was seventeen, I believe, because her family in St. Louis was not doing well financially and her father (Fred Pilates—Joe's brother) asked Joe if she could come to NY and live with him. Once she got there Joe and Clara immediately began teaching her the exercises and she became a studio assistant and worked for them. It was not clear to me whether she worked for room and board or whether they actually paid her as well. I do remember that a member of the audience asked her, 'How do you pronounce the name?' Her response brought the crowd to laughter and cheers when she stated: 'Well, we always said *pilots*.' She said that she still did her exercises almost every day and got down on the floor and went right into *the hundred* without a warm up—all 83 years of her—and then proceeded to roll up and roll over and the crowd went nuts!"

www.parklandpilates.com

Jay Grimes with more than forty years of Pilates experience, got his start in Pilates by training with Joseph Pilates during the last few years of Joseph's life, and then with Joseph's wife Clara following Joseph's death. Jay began teaching in the original 8th Ave studio in New York, then moved with the studio to 56th Street where he taught alongside (as well as studied with) Romana Kryzanowska & John Winters. He has made numerous TV appearances, including the Discovery Channel's Fit TV with Marilu Henner, with whom he also made videos for her Body Victory program. A professional dancer for eighteen years, Jay attributes his injury free dancing career to pilates. Jay compares the idea of a well tuned body with a wonderfully maintained musical instrument—if an instrument is tuned and in good working order it can be used to play any type or style of music well. Our body is the same way, according to Jay—a well tuned body doesn't care if it's bowling or dancing ballet.

Peter Fiasca, who studied with Jay calls him, ". . . another extraordinary 1st generation teacher."

www.jaygrimes.com

These are the people who have ushered in Joe Pilates' method, and kept it alive as a practice that transforms lives and transcends fitness trends. By taking a moment to honor these visionaries, it is my hope that their inspiration will live on in the new generation of Pilates teachers and students as we move through the challenges of the 21st century.

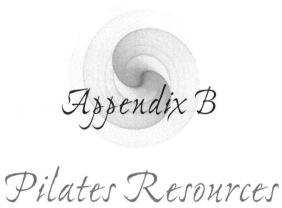

Appendix B

Pilates Resources

Here are some distinctive Pilates organizations, teaching institutions and equipment manufacturers that foster these principles and values in step with 21st century needs.

Websites are added to further the readers need to know more.

Pilates Organizations
The Pilates Method Alliance (PMA) a not for profit organization

The Pilates method has been in continuous use in the United States since 1926 when its creator Joseph Pilates and his wife Clara immigrated to New York City from Germany. The Pilates Method Alliance (PMA) is the international not for profit professional association for the Pilates method. The PMA's mission is to protect the public by establishing certification and continuing education standards for Pilates professionals.

The PMA made history in 2005 by launching the first industry wide certification exam for the Pilates method in the United States. The PMA has established recommended industry performance parameters guiding the practice of all PMA Certified and non-certified Pilates teachers to further bring professionalism to Pilates.

The PMA is well aware that as Pilates exercise has gained popularity, confusion and controversy have increased in the media, the public and even between Pilates teachers. Since the PMA's goal is protect and enhance the Pilates method, and introduce it to public schools fulfilling on a vision of Joseph Pilates—shaping the fitness ideals of our next generation, it is necessary to establish a position statement to clarify the perception of what Pilates was historically and what it is today.

www.pilatesmethodalliance.org

The United States Pilates Association™ (U.S.P.A.™)

U.S.P.A. honors the legacy of Joseph Pilates' teachings, mind/body wellness philosophy, and is committed to preserving and promoting his original message of vibrant health, quality of life, and his unwavering dedication to excellence.

The U.S.P.A.™ is home of the New York Pilates Studio® Teacher Certification Program and provides Teacher Training, Certification and Continuing Education in Authentic Pilates™, as well as Authentic Pilates™ Education to the public and private sectors.

In addition to Teacher Certification and Education, the U.S.P.A.™ is working on new outreach programs which will include public schools, hospitals, rehabilitation centers, and specialized programs for the elderly, disabled, and learning challenged populations. Joseph Pilates envisioned that his methodology would benefit people of all ages and all body types.

www.unitedstatespilatesassociation.com

Physical Mind Institute (The Method Pilates)

The Method Pilates is the name associated with the evolution of The Method which is what clients called Joe's work when he was alive. Eve Gentry, his first teacher, taught for him until his death in 1967 and the following year she moved to Santa Fe and opened up a Pilates Studio on Camino de la Luz. This began the first evolution of the technique which was refined in 1991 when Eve and others—including all those now called The Elders—Ron Fletcher, Romana, Bruce King, Carola Trier, Kathy Grant, Mary Bowen—were part of the first Advisory Board of the Institute for the Pilates Method. Later, in 1996 when the Institute's name was changed to Physical Mind Institute, a new group of advisors participated as part of the Working Board which included Rael Isacovitz, Amy Alpers, Jillian Hessel, Michele Larsson, Karma Kinszler, Deborah Lessen. Today another team ensures continued growth of The Method. This evolution of the work that Joe created almost a century ago is what we believe he would have undertaken had he lived into the 21st Century.

www.themethodpilates.com

Teaching Institutions

The Pilates Center

The Pilates Center, located in Boulder, Colorado, was established in 1990 by sisters Amy Taylor Alpers and Rachel Taylor Segel. The sisters trained in New York City at The Pilates Studio and were certified by Romana Kryzanowska, heir to the classical tradition of Joseph Pilates.

In 1991, The Pilates Center established their Teacher Training Program. Developed with the assistance of Romana Kryzanowska and Steve Giordano.

Their mission is to heal the world by empowering people to transform their health and 'Return to Life'.

www.thepilatescenter.com

Polestar Pilates

Polestar Pilates is an international community of research-oriented movement science professionals, transferring advanced knowledge to our clients to improve health and well-being, through the application of Pilates and various methodologies of movement science.

The Polestar curriculum is based on Pilates principles—not exercise repertoire alone. This enables Polestar practitioners to create exercise programs to address the needs of special populations (golfers, tennis players, dancers, etc.).

Polestar's vision is to Impact the world through intelligent movement, which fosters awareness of self and community.

www.polestarpilates.com

Classical Pilates

Classical Pilates mission is to preserve Joseph Pilates' traditional method of mental and physical conditioning through teaching, continuing education, and instructional materials. This work is presented in the award winning *Classical Pilates Technique* DVDs, demonstrating a progression of safe but challenging workouts for the entire body and mind. The critically acclaimed companion book, *Discovering Pure Classical Pilates*, traces the history and philosophy of Joseph Pilates, differentiating his method from derivative approaches. Pure Classical Pilates workshops promote a deeper understanding of the traditional work and the Academy Directory provides a comprehensive list of classically trained teachers.

www.classicalpilates.net

BASI Pilates (Body Arts and Science International)

BASI Pilates™ (Body Arts and Science International™) was formed in 1989 by world-renowned Pilates educator, Rael Isacowitz. BASI Pilates™ is a true blending of the Art and Science of human movement, relating specifically to the works of Joseph H. Pilates. BASI Pilates™ honors and preserves the legacy of Joseph and Clara Pilates: presenting the original principles and repertoire (utilizing all the Pilates equipment), at the same time integrating contemporary scientific developments and evolution of the method.

It is an educational vehicle, which upholds the standards of the work of Joseph Pilates and teaches the essence of his philosophy. Well being is the ultimate goal, and in pursuit of this goal every level of the human condition will be addressed to better each individual as well as the world we live in. No person shall be denied this privilege. BASI Pilates™ endeavors to grow in substance, not only in size, and will always strive to be true to science, to knowledge, to artistry and to the intentions of Joseph Pilates in providing the finest education possible!

www.basipilates.com

Power Pilates

Power Pilates is distinguished in the industry by an unwavering emphasis on training that honors the integrity of the original method developed by Joseph Pilates.

Whether you visit our flagship studios in New York City and Westchester, travel to one of our of global training centers, or take a class from a Power Pilates trained instructor at your local fitness center—you are guaranteed to receive an consistent, classically-based, invigorating and fitness focused Pilates workout

At Power Pilates—our students discover a profound sense of community. At its roots, Power Pilates has sought to create a Pilates community in the spirit of Joseph Pilates—energetic, committed and ever evolving. The founders of Power Pilates, started with a nascent group of studio instructors, have since propelled the total population of Power Pilates professionals and consumers into thousands upon thousands on a global scale

www.powerpilates.com

Peak Pilates

At Peak Pilates®, we've always been committed to preserving the integrity and genius of Joseph H. Pilates. Today, his singular method of exercise has re-emerged powerfully to help today's fitness enthusiasts and athletes achieve new levels of performance. At Peak Pilates, we're delivering that excitement in new ways with the advanced equipment, education and execution techniques you need to create a competitive edge in life and business.

Peak Pilates® offers premier education in a flexible schedule that's right for you. Our students have access to a full range of classes—from workshops to teacher training certification programs. Our classical philosophy is simple: We teach how to teach and not just what to teach. Classical Pilates is rhythmic, fluid and focused—connecting one movement to the next to build greater strength, flexibility and endurance, and our coaching model heightens each trainee's confidence and capability as an instructor.

www.peakpilates.com

Pilates Equipment Manufacturers

Balanced Body

Balanced Body is the world's largest manufacturer of Pilates equipment. The company was the first to substantially update Joseph Pilates' equipment with state-of-the-art engineering, materials and technology. Ken Endelman, the company's founder and owner, has designed hundreds of improvements to Pilates' original equipment, many of which have since become industry standards. Balanced Body has been awarded twenty-five U.S. patents, and numerous foreign patents for his inventions, with more patents pending. Formerly known as Current Concepts, the company changed its name to Balanced Body in 1999.Our mission is to enhance people's lives by providing mind-body fitness products that set the industry standards for innovation, safety, craftsmanship, efficiency and beauty.

Balanced Body University a subdivision of Balanced Body offers unique educational formats including a mentoring program for aspiring professionals called *Passing the Torch*. This program was created to help shape the next generation of leaders in the Pilates community. It was inspired by a discussion with Lolita San Miguel in the fall of 2008. "Passing the Torch Mentoring Program" is a master's program designed for Pilates instructors who have been teaching Pilates for many years and long for a deepening of their work through a mentorship program with a first or second generation teacher.

www.pilates.com

Gratz Pilates Equipment

Gratz is the original manufacturer of Pilates apparatus and the industry's established source for authentic equipment. Our New York City custom fabrication shop has been in business since 1929, crafting not only Joseph Pilates' unique design, but also museum-quality furniture, architectural metal, and sculpture for many of the world's greatest designers.

Over a half century ago, our company's patriarch Frank Gratz applied his engineering and metalwork expertise while working with Joseph Pilates. Frank's son Donald continued this commitment to preserving the integrity of their apparatus and in the late 1960's collaborated with Romana Kryzanowska as she carried on the Pilates legacy. Thanks to these relationships, Gratz has maintained a fidelity to Pilates' original vision by fabricating apparatus with unerring craftsmanship and exacting specifications.

While Gratz is located in New York City, our equipment can be found in studios worldwide. Teachers and students know the Gratz difference and consider our apparatus an indispensable part of their practice and we are proud to carry on the tradition and serve the Pilates community. You can count on Gratz to protect Joseph Pilates' vision by respecting the details of every item we produce.

www.gratz-pilates.com

Stott Pilates Equipment

STOTT PILATES® is a contemporary approach to the original exercise method pioneered by the late Joseph Pilates. Co-founders Moira and Lindsay G. Merrithew, along with a team of physical therapists, sports medicine and fitness professionals, have spent more than two decades refining the STOTT PILATES method of exercise and equipment. This resulted in the inclusion of modern principles of exercise science and spinal rehabilitation, making it one of the safest and effective methods available. This clear and detailed approach forms the basis for STOTT PILATES training and certification programs. It's used by rehab and prenatal clients, athletes, celebrities and everyone in between. We're the largest full-service organization in the world providing cutting-edge Pilates education, Pilates equipment, and Pilates DVDs. Your one-stop-shop for quality mind-body fitness. Experience Pilates for a lifetime with us.

www.stottpilates.com

Root Pilates Equipment

Root's goal is to be the premier source of Pilates equipment and to continually elevate the standards for function, quality of craftsmanship, and durability. True to our roots and the Pilates Method our mission is: to provide the Pilates teacher and the enthusiast with the very best equipment and support.

Root was born out of our drive to create products using quality design, construction and eco-friendly materials. With over a decade as one of the country's largest manufacturers of Pilates equipment, Root incorporates extensive client feedback in producing an exquisitely crafted iteration of the classic Joseph Pilates design. Using modern materials selected for durability and performance, Root fulfills the demand of discriminating teachers for a product that will provide a superior experience in the studio environment. Root is a unique culture . . . a blend of people with lifelong backgrounds in woodworking, engineering, metal craft, upholstery, and Pilates technique. It is a culture of continuous improvement for our equipment, our customers, and our environment. At Root we employ methods, which minimize our impact on the environment. In addition to recycling, using sustainable materials, and reducing our energy demand, we reduce VOC emissions by utilizing waterborne lacquers and powder-coated finishes. Our equipment utilizes the finest sustainable materials available. Bamboo, Northern Red Oak, and Hard Maple are sourced from suppliers who use sustainable forestry practices. Stainless steel poles are extremely durable and eliminate the need for the toxic plating process used in chroming. Finally, Root equipment is hand crafted with meticulous care to last a lifetime.

www.rootmfg.com

Recommended Reading

For those interested in reading about 'how to do' Pilates at home, here are a few books that are well illustrated and will lead you through the Pilates mat work:

The Pilates Body . . . by Brooke Siler

Pilates Body in Motion . . . By Alycea Ungaro

The Everything Pilates Book . . . by Amy Taylor Alpers and Rachel Taylor Segel

The Pilates Method of Physical and Mental Conditioning . . . Philip Friedman and Gail Eisen

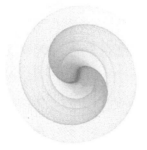

Letter to the Reader

Dear Reader,

The resolve you may find in this book is not a panacea. The inner work we all come to do in our lifetime and the myriad of paths it may take—the "archeological digs" we perform on ourselves—is necessarily subjective. I am not that pragmatic in defining life or a return to it . . . nor do I believe in all doctrine. Believe what you will through conscious reason and that includes what you glean from this book.

I came to trust my inner journey to uncover what I know as my truth. Nothing can substitute for or equal this experience. The inception of the idea for this book—inspired by selective research and personal stories contained within—simply made sense to me.

Each of us has a particular structure to our psyche. According to Carl Gustav Jung a Swiss psychiatrist who fathered the theory of a' collective unconscious 'shared by all human beings, described in Jungian Typology, we all know and experience life through what Jung called 4 "functions:" Thinking and Feeling which are opposites (one will be in the conscious, the other in the unconscious) and Sensation and Intuition (again one in the conscious, the other in the unconscious). My conscious 1st Function is Feeling. And my 2nd Function, also consciously available, is Sensation (the body, the physical and manifest world). This is how I was born. This has been my comfortable approach to deciphering the world.

Then crossing the threshold of mid-life at about forty-five, a change occurs for each of us which continues onward to the end. Our 3rd and 4th unconscious functions push up for development. For me my 3rd function is Intuition and my 4th is Thinking. From my intuition and thinking functions I have written this book.

Our greatest teacher is the 4th function. It is the hardest to reach—resistant—requiring heroic patience and perseverance to access and develop from. This is the root of our creativity and the root of our unique contribution and personal authority. This 4th function is also importantly the opening presence of our spirit—spirit emerging in form. This book has been born from my intuition bridging into my thinking. To some I may seem to over-spiritualize the pioneering efforts brought forth by Joe and Clara and that the effect it has on our lives is more qualitative in its residual energetic essence than the act of doing Pilates itself. I am told by those who knew them that they were very down to earth sensate people, not questing as I certainly am. Perhaps we get as much as we put into what we do. It may not be the thing itself but rather the projecting of ourselves into whatever our passion and interest is that creates the spirit and the transformation. If this is so, it diminishes nothing for me of the importance of Pilates in my life, or in the personal stories recounted of others in this book and countless others "out there and all around the world." It is now as Joe and Clara had hoped and envisioned it would be. Pilates is world-wide.

To further support you in your contemplations, discussions, understanding, and incorporation of these ideas into your life and work, I invite you, individually, or others, as a group, to contact me so that I may speak with you in either the reading of this book or your work with Pilates. I can be reached at Gary@pilatespathtohealth.com or (970) 263-8700.

In good health,

Gary Calderone/ Edited by Mary Bowen, Pilates Elder and Jungian Analyst

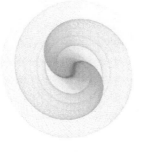

Acknowledgments

The inception of this book, and its development, was directed by something higher and wiser than myself. More so, this book was birthed by a village of supporters, nurturers and believers, whom without, what you hold in your hand, would not have come into the world. Thanks to:

- Michael Lindemann who insisted I am a writer and taught me how.

- Stephanie Anderson for believing whole heartedly in what I was doing and supporting me through the thick and thin of this process. Without her diligence in her Pilates practice and gracious 'seed money', this book would not have come into existence.

- Mark Anderson for reviving my ailing heart and restoring my health.

- Wendy Leblanc-Arbuckle from the day we met to the magical moment you asked me to join you on your Pilates journey in Austin. Your unconditional love is indescribably mystical and your passion to help shift the human condition, one person and one thought at a time, has led me here.

- Michael Arbuckle for the day you held the space for me to step into the 'conversation'. I am more now than I thought I could ever be. Your 'heart of hearts', relentless integrity, monetary wisdom, and support throughout my process is greatly appreciated and duly noted.

- Peter and Cathy Ulrich for their ground work in the beginnings of Concepts in Contrology and the fabulous dinners, the bottles of wine, and all the laughs which provided a supportive, creative space for us to venture in.

- Don Huss for your friendship, belief, vision, and generous financial assistance.

- Mim Neal for your unyielding trust by inviting me into your circle of health care providers and your generous financial assistance.

- Mary Bowen who allowed my voice to come through her wisdom to redefine the greater gift Pilates offers humanity.

- My family: Gene Calderone, Rose Calderone, Tom Calderone, and Mary Letizia, for all their unconditional love, monetary support, and relentless belief that one day I'll make it!

- Rebecca Adams, your 'healing touch' goes a long way.

- Susie Harrison, for believing in us, still, after the fact, and supporting what we originally set out to do. I love you, eternally.

- Peter Anthony, my soul brother who shines his light and illuminates my path, dissolving what appears to be darkness and despair. Your unsurpassed consciousness and creativity to awaken the world inspires me.

- Mya, our dog, for her unconditional love, when there was nothing left to hold on to.

- Sebastian Posern my dear friend and great healer who got me back on my feet. Literally! And your financial support.

- Renee Hawkis for generously offering your service to intervene when I had lost my footing in the world.

- Susan St. Clair for cheering on my vision and making me laugh at the obvious.

- Steve Finnestead and Roxanne Storlie for being there since the beginning of my work, culminating in this book. Truly, without their endless hours of help, this book, nor I, would have made it this far.

- Michael and Wendy Arbuckle for your generous financial support.

- Rachael Ananda for keeping me on track with the stars and planets aligning for my higher good.

- Judy Basow for being the best salesperson in uncharted territory.

- Elizabeth Kittrell you are the keeper of my sanity. Your wisdom and heart has opened more doors to understanding, compassion, and grace than I have ever known.

- Heidi Miller for always whispering into me a reminder of who I really am, and for caretaking my energetic state.

- Toni D. Holm, Publisher and George E. Tice, Managing Editor for putting up with me 'kicking and screaming' in keeping their commitment to their noble mission with an uncommon sense of listening for the readers' needs and uncanny timing for when the book was really, really, no really ready. Saying thank you just isn't enough! (Sending you both to the South of France may be in order!)

- To the Word Keepers, Inc. intuitive publishing team: Laura Daniels, my Copyeditor who captured my voice with such clarity that even I am moved by its message; Shannon Hassan, Development Editor who took the time to listen to my journey and greatly enhanced the distinction that allows the reader to step into the message this book offers; David Dalton, initial Art Director who creatively brought design to both book cover and interior design sample chapters; and to the production team of 1106 Design, LLC, who brought the finishing touches to the full book cover and the revises to the book's interior final pages. I'm grateful to have had a talented, caring staff managing the health of the book.

- To the early Word Keepers, Inc. Reader Reviewers, thank you! Your reviews gave back a million-fold in the development process of my book: Tom Calderone, Carmen Mendoza, Carole Balawender, Bob Schneider, Toni Wolf, Kristen Fairgrieve, Sandra Smiley, Diane Hower, Regan Windsor, Laura Ussery, and Joshua McDaniel.

- To the Pilates Professional reviewers, I'm deeply indebted for your gracious time, energy, and valuable feedback: Ashley Robinson, Joyce Yost Ulrich, Zoe Stein Pierce, Ann Arnoult, Pat Guyton, Clare Dunphy, Jennifer Zimann &

Mathew, Andria Davisson, Lara Kolesar, Marguerite Ogle, Rachael Taylor-Segel, Gerald N. Morigerato, Heidi Miller, Serene Calkins, Jebidiah Gorham, Maila Rider, Nan Feist, Melissa Macourek, and Brent Anderson.

- The staff, faculty and clients of The Pilates Center, The Pilates Center of Fort Collins, and The Pilates Center of Austin for tolerating my enthusiasm through my formidable years of gestation.

- Maila Blossom Rider for dedicating her time and energy to a cause she has supported since the onset.

- Sean Anderson whose courageous journey into himself makes transformation tangible and taught me volumes about what is possible.

- Lee Cooper for your relentless enthusiasm for life and the work.

- Abby Bloedorn for being a torch bearer of Pilates as a greater cause of health.

- Laura Ussery for your ability to trust the process, listen internally, and claim what is possible and apply that 'felt sense' to living a life you love.

- David and Laura Ussery for your financial support.

All my Pilates teachers, too numerous to list (you know who you are), I couldn't have done this without your service to the betterment of my health. Special acknowledgement and a resounding heartfelt shout of recognition for the quality of attention the following teachers brought into my awareness, when I couldn't find it within, goes out to:

- Amy Alpers, Rachel Segel, Steve Giordano, Romana Kryzanowska, Debra Kolwey, Amy Lange, and Lisa Csillan-McAleavy.

- Wendy Leblanc-Arbuckle, Lara Kolesar, Susie Haggas, and Cara Reeser.

Special Thanks . . . to Brent Anderson for keeping the global vision of Pilates work and the impact it can have, for standing in a greater cause, holding the space for possibility to reign through 'whole being health' and illuminating this notion across oceans and continents, "By heightening our awareness of self through Pilates, we heighten our awareness of our influence of others, which can lead to a glimpse of reality and the hopeful global shift towards peace, one Pilates Enthusiast at a time."

SPECIAL ACKNOWLEDGMENT: Mary Bowen, Wendy Leblanc-Arbuckle, and Michael Arbuckle . . . there are not words to express my deepest gratitude, only the joy my heart feels when I read what you breathed into the life of this book. For all the time, energy, and wisdom you bestowed, standing up for the transformational distinction this book can offer its collective readership through clarity, grace, *and a deeper insight beyond the movement.* Because of you, this book is a marker, a signpost pointing the way along the worn path of all who came before and all who will continue the journey of the Pilates legacy. The affirmation it will have on the global community, lending credence, as a resource for future generations of Pilates teachers who value their work as more than delivering exercises, I am deeply grateful.

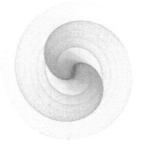

About the Author

G ary Calderone was lecturing in three countries, immersed in holistic health sciences prior to his Pilates experience, setting the stage for this book to be written. His dedication and exploration of the Pilates Method, as it relates to the experience of a series of exercises, engagement in body/ mind/spirit connection, and overall health and balance, comes out of 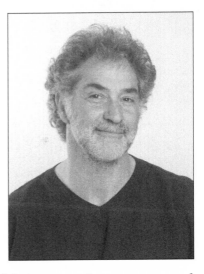 that immersion and his history of injury and recovery and personal need. He continues to benefit from his own experiences with the Pilates Method from the positions of student and teacher.

Gary is a second-generation teacher, originating and graduating from the Pilates Center in Boulder, Colorado, in 1993. During that year, as founding Director of the Pilates Center of Fort Collins, Colorado, Gary brought the classical teaching to the attention of the medical community, illuminating the healing potential of Pilates, particularly around chronic/acute patient populations, culminating in collaboration with the Brain Injury Recovery Program (BIRP), to enhance patient recovery.

During 2000 and 2001 Gary went on to complete eighteen months of transformational training as a protégé of Wendy Leblanc-Arbuckle, creator of the Core Connections® Pilates 3-Core Body Mapping Perspective at The Pilates Center of Austin (PCA. Inspired by his own training, his life altering experiences, and the inspirational benefits of training others, Gary integrated his own philosophy and understanding of the power and practicality of the Pilates Method for a healthy, holistic approach to life.

In 2003 'Concepts in Contrology: Going Beyond Technique' was presented at the Pilates Method Alliance 3rd Annual International Conference, 'Pilates Pure and Simple,' in Denver, Colorado. In 2004 Gary was a featured speaker at the Polestar Pilates 3rd Annual International Conference, 'The World of Pilates Excellence' in Miami, Florida. At the Polestar event, in addition to his featured talk, Gary led a roundtable forum on 'The Relevance of Pilates in the 21st Century.' Gary continues to present his work to Pilates enthusiasts nationally and internationally.

At a personal and professional level, Gary lives and teaches from his understanding that the practice of the Pilates Method is more than just an exercise regimen. "People are seeking balance in all categories of their lives. My hope is that my book is timely in providing readers access to a deeper level of personal care in their own path to health by recognizing how Pilates continues to adapt and serve the needs of a global community—now, in this 21st century more than ever."

His professional memberships include: The Institute of Noetic Sciences (IONS), The International Society for the Study of Subtle Energies and Energy Medicine (ISSSEEM), and completion of and continued participation in The Landmark Education Curriculum for Living.

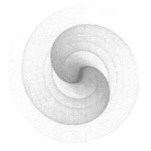

Applause

"Gary Calderone and I first met many years ago and realized that we had a very strong connection in the aspect of Pilates embracing a philosophy of whole being health, incorporating the spiritual and mental components of Joseph Pilates' philosophy and lifestyle. Calderone has done an amazing job of capturing the essence of Joe's work in his new book The Pilates Path to Health: Body, Mind, and Spirit. This must read is a significant addition to the limited library of the work enjoyed my millions around the globe. Calderone's insightful recount of 'Contrology' brings awareness to vital aspects of our health as individuals and as a society. By heightening our awareness of self through Pilates, we heighten our awareness of our influence of others, which can lead to a glimpse of reality and the hopeful global shift towards peace one Pilates Enthusiast at a time.

It is minds like Calderone's mind that will help speed up the day, where a critical mass will embrace a peaceful and balanced state between mind, body, and spirit hastening the shift in our world's paradigm from one of anger to one of love. The beauty of Calderone's book is his ability to make it personal and write it so that everyone can enjoy the deeper benefits that are associated with this great work that we all love and has changed our lives as admirers, enthusiasts, and teachers of Pilates. Great work, Gary!!!"

—Brent D. Anderson, PT, Ph.D., OCS, President of Polestar Pilates

"I have known Gary for twenty years; he is one of the first graduates of The Pilates Center Teacher Training Program and learned directly from Romana, as well as Amy and myself. He has been passionate about the Pilates method since his first lesson and this book is the latest expression of his long-held dream to share the wonders of Pilates with the world.

Because there is so much trendy hype about Pilates it is imperative that the real value of this work be spoken about loudly and creatively as Gary has done in this book. Pilates is transformative. We teachers are blessed with the experience of taking victims of terrible pain and re-forming them into powerful, pain free activists with a zest for living. In partnership with our clients we help them not only effect powerful transformations in their bodies but in their mental states, watching reclusive, angry individuals grow empathetic and giving, shifting into delighting in their lives and the world, being able to participate actively in making a difference in their own lives but also the lives of others. As Gary describes so richly, the power of Pilates is so profound it can motivate them to change the deepest patterns of their lives and then touch those around them newly.

This book shares much of the truth of Joseph Pilates' method and aligns it with other great modern thinkers to bring it into the 21st century."

—Rachel Taylor Segel with **Amy Alpers,** Co-founder and
Co-owner The Pilates Center, Boulder, Colorado

"There are many books on the market that describe the Pilates method in detail and precision. However, Pilates is not just another workout fad. Joseph Pilates' message is a profound commitment to the life well lived. Health is a balance of the body, mind, and spirit. These are the essential elements for happiness and success. Gary Calderone has applied his study and life to the embodiment of the Pilates philosophy, reminding the reader that Pilates is more than an exercise regimen; it is a path of study and enlightenment."

—Pat Guyton, PMA Certified Pilates Teacher™,
Pat Guyton Pilates, Inc., Pilates Conservatory®

"Gary asks the right questions, inviting us to think outside the box about living a balanced life through the practice of Pilates. He masterfully unlocks the essence of Pilates' greatest secret—why and how Pilates profoundly impacts both student and teacher, weaving threads from other disciplines to confirm their universal connection. He illuminates the truth about how choices for our inner health are mirrored in the manifestation of our outer experience, thereby strengthening global consciousness. Truly inspiring!"

—**Clare Dunphy,** Peak Pilates Master Trainer,
Director, Progressive Bodyworks, Inc.

"Gary Calderone's new book The Pilates Path to Health: Body, Mind, and Spirit *has made me more excited than ever about this wonderful work that I practice and teach. He breathes new life into Joseph Pilates' own book* Return to Life *and gives the reader the perspective to appreciate the gift and potential impact of Contrology that was given to the world."*

—**Joyce Yost Ulrich,** PMA® Certified Pilates Teacher,
Yamuna Body Rolling™ Practitioner, Owner, Pilates Treehouse

"Gary has done an amazing job of writing about inspirational, almost esoteric, ideas while keeping them tagged into earth and woven with real-life experience. He has thrown the door wide open for an important conversation about how Pilates connects us to personal transformation and positive global change."

—**Marguerite Ogle,** the guide to Pilates at About.com.

"This book is relevant and necessary for our future and our evolutionary process. This is a service to humanity, a fertilizer for personal growth and ultimate utopian awakening. Gary's writing and his experience is authentic; he gives you a telescope glimpse of a better way to live. Gary outlines our human challenges and provides tools for rising above those inner conflicts with Pilates as the vehicle. He meets the paradox moments

with compassion and strength. It is so simply sophisticated, honestly written with details and experiences that make you hungry to feel it in your body."

—**Maila Blossom Rider**/Pilates, Yoga and Franklin method professional/Owner of the Pilates Yoga Company, Windsor, Colorado

"The Pilates Path to Health: Body, Mind, and Spirit by Gary Calderone is a timely contribution to literature in the Health, Fitness and Wellness industry. Gary's ability to present the material in a reader-friendly format with compelling evidence intertwined should be applauded. Our industry is consistently seeking new models for the delivery of integrated and results-focused initiatives that provide for the healthy lifestyles and outcomes of our clients. The Pilates approach to health truly focuses on awareness, choice, and results. As an industry leader I believe this book will add value to the industry understanding of Pilates and its multifaceted benefits. Gary's writing illustrates his passion for why he and others practice and teach Pilates. **The Pilates Path to Health** *provides evidence of the restorative health benefits for those who consciously choose the Pilates Method."*

—**Jeb Gorham,** Ph.D., Wellness Director—Central Manager Miramont Lifestyle Fitness, Former Director of Education Peak Pilates

". . . An inspiring guide to optimal human vitality and balanced living. Gary Calderone expands the definition of 'fitness' in his quest to understand the mission of Joseph Pilates and the profound results of his work."

—**Matthew Zumann,** CPT, Structural Therapist—
Jennifer Golden Zumann, CPT, Medicinal Herbalist
(Co-Owners of Pilates Chicago, Inc.)

"This book is a wonderful support for individuals on a path of understanding themselves through the practice of the Pilates Method. Gary's writing illuminates aspects of these practices that transform body, mind, and spirit. In an age when Pilates mainstream popularity and easy access cause the

loss of these vitals elements, it is necessary for strong voices, like this voice, to be heard, so that the depth of the Pilates Method and what it can offer the practitioner are not lost."

—**Melissa Macourek,** Samsara Pilates

"Finally a book on the Pilates Method that is a not a 'how-to' but a 'why.' Gary's book speaks to our common love of the work and the amazing power of change that we all see every day in our practice. This book takes me back to before the copyright days when the creative differences were celebrated and there was an amazing unified feeling of how special Joseph Pilates' method was and how blessed we were to be a part of that vision. We know how cool this work is and how great it feels. Gary does a good job of attempting to define this nature of the work."

—**Nan Feist,** LMP, Pilates Instructor, Somatic Educator

"As we move another generation away from the elders, it is more important than ever that we take the time and attention to teach our clients and mentor the new instructors how to receive 'the priceless gift of physical well-being, mental calm, and spiritual peace' through mindful Pilates practice."

—**Serene Rene Calkins,** P.T.